TERESA SHIELDS PARKER

# SWEET FREEDOM

## LOSING WEIGHT AND KEEPING IT OFF WITH GOD'S HELP

*"Let me be clear, the Anointed One has set us free—
not partially, but completely and wonderfully free!
We must always cherish this truth and stubbornly
refuse to go back into the bondage of our past"*

Galatians 5:1 TPT

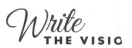

# SWEET FREEDOM
## LOSING WEIGHT AND KEEPING IT OFF WITH GOD'S HELP

Printed in the USA

ISBN: 978-0-9910012-5-5      Print

Library of Congress Control Number: 2016901976

Published by Write the Vision | Columbia, Missouri    *Write* THE VISION.NET

Scripture taken from the *Amplified®* Bible is marked AMP. Copyright © 2015 by The Lockman Foundation. All rights reserved. Used by permission.

Scripture taken from *The Message ®* is marked MSG. Copyright © 1993, 1994, 1995, 1996, 2000, 2001, 2002. Used by permission of NavPress Publishing Group. Colorado Springs, CO. All rights reserved.

Scripture is taken from God's Word®, is marked GW. Copyright © 1995 God's Word to the Nations. Used by permission of Baker Publishing Group.

Scripture taken from the *New American Standard Bible®* is marked NASB. Copyright © 1960, 1962, 1963, 1968, 1971, 1972, 1973, 1975, 1977, 1995 by The Lockman Foundation. Used by permission.

Scripture taken from the *Holy Bible New International Version ®* is marked NIV. Copyright © 1973, 1978, 1984, 2011 Biblica. Used by permission of Zondervan. All rights reserved.

Scripture taken from the *New King James Version* of the Bible is marked NKJV. Copyright © 1982 by Thomas Nelson, Inc. Used by permission. All rights reserved.

Scripture taken from the *Holy Bible, New Living Translation* is marked NLT. Copyright © 1996, 2004, 2007, 2913. Used by permission of Tyndale House Publishers, Inc., Wheaton, Illinois. All rights reserved.

Scripture taken from *The Living Bible* is marked TLB. Copyright © 1971 by Tyndale House Foundation. Used by permission of Tyndale House Publishers Inc., Carol Stream, Illinois 60188. All rights reserved. The Living Bible, TLB, and the The Living Bible logo are registered trademarks of Tyndale House Publishers.

Scripture taken from *John: Eternal Love, The Passion Translation* ™ is marked TPT. Copyright © 2014. Used by permission of 5 Fold Media, LLC, Syracuse, NY 13039, United States of America. All rights reserved.

Scripture taken from *Proverbs: Wisdom from Above, The Passion Translation* ™ is marked TPT. Copyright © 2013. Used by permission of 5 Fold Media, LLC, Syracuse, NY 13039, United States of America. All rights reserved.

Scripture taken from *Letters from Heaven by the Apostle Paul, The Passion Translation* ™ is marked TPT. Copyright © 2013. Used by permission of 5 Fold Media, LLC, Syracuse, NY 13039, United States of America. All rights reserved.

To Contact the Author:

# www.TeresaShieldsParker.com

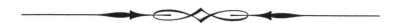

This book is for anyone who is serious about overcoming struggles with food and weight. Teresa candidly shares her brave journey of overcoming the emotional, psychological, and spiritual issues that kept her trapped in a vicious cycle of addiction and shame.

Through her journey you will learn how to invite God to lovingly and practically guide you every step of the way. And, you will be encouraged and inspired to choose life and pursue your recovery at any cost.

**—Dr. Margaret Nagib**
Clinical Psychologist & Eating Disorders Specialist,
Timberline Knolls Residential Treatment Center
Director, Bethel Sozo for Professional Counselors
Founder, TheDunamisProject.org

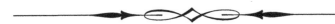

am excited that you made the decision to read and learn from this book. It will change your whole life! *Sweet Freedom* is the story of one woman's discovery of the power of God in her and the true meaning of victory over difficulties and depression.

As you read her story you, too, will learn how to overcome the many psychological and spiritual problems that plague our modern age. Teresa Shields Parker's journey into wholeness and maturity can also be your guide to discovering and embracing your true identity.

I know millions of people around the world can and will find new life as they read this book. I want you to be one of these people. As you read *Sweet Freedom* and apply the principles it teaches, you will find the real you and the real God inside the authentic you!

**—Joan Hunter**
Author/Evangelist
Founder and President of Joan Hunter Ministries

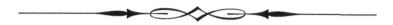

Teresa has written a book that gives the path to freedom on every page. True freedom is found not in our strength, but in the strength of the Strength-Giver Jesus Christ.

Jesus came to set the captives free, and He offers freedom to all who will put their trust in Him.

Teresa points the reader to the truth of God's Word, and the freedom found when we obey the way He leads. Those who have a little or a lot of weight to lose will find help in the pages of this book.

Teresa's honesty and transparency draw us in and give us hope.

**—Carole Lewis**
Director Emeritus, First Place 4 Health
Author of *Give God A Year, Change Your Life Forever*

SWEET FREEDOM

# ACKNOWLEDGEMENTS

There are many who have helped me bring this book to you. I am grateful to those who willingly give their talents and gifts to help me use mine. It is always hard to know where to begin to thank people.

A special shout out goes to those who read, proofed and edited *Sweet Freedom*. These include my awesome team: Shannon Fox, Marilyn Logan, Karen Fritzemeier, Michelle Smith, Rhonda Burrows, Mary Jennie Bodard, Linda Ordway and many in *Sweet Freedom* Book Launch Group. Thanks, too, for your suggestions, positive comments and encouraging words.

To the ones who are always my first readers, my sister, Renee Shields Allen, and my brother, Mark Randall Shields, thanks for loving me no matter what I write. Thanks to my aunt, Joyce Smith, who is always the voice of reason and reassurance.

Coaches turned friends are the best kind of coaches. Thanks for being both, Aida Ingram, Russ Hardesty and Wendy K. Walters. Of course, no book of mine is ever complete without a Wendy Walters cover.

I could not have completed this book and the study guide without the steady vigilance of the "watchmen on my wall".[1]

The 23 faithful members of TSP Prayer Group prayed whenever I sent a request. Many prayed at special times for the book, for its contents, its title and for you, the readers. I will never undertake writing a book without a dedicated prayer team.

A special thanks to Sweet Change Weight Loss Coaching Group, you are my inspiration. You, and all those who want to be set free of food addictions, are why I keep doing what I do.

Special thanks to my son, Andrew Parker, for keeping all my technology running and answering my crazy computer questions day or night. Thanks to my daughter and son-in-law, Jenny and Nigel Church, who both should be writing books and will one day. Just knowing you believe in me, even though you're far away, helps.

My deepest thanks goes to my husband, Roy Parker, who can make all my anxieties, fears, doubts and misgivings go away with his understanding and gentle, loving ways.

Above all, thanks to God Almighty who reminds me daily it was for freedom that I was set free.

ENDNOTES

1.  1 Isaiah 62:6 NLT

# D E D I C A T I O N

*In honor of my parents,*
*Ernest and Donna Shields.*

*To Dad:*

*Thanks for showing me intentional devotion*
*to God brings rewards most people, even*
*Christians, can't even begin to fathom.*

*To Mom:*

*Thanks for showing me through your life that*
*no matter how much bondage I may feel I*
*am in, sweet freedom is just a prayer away.*

*Thank you both for being overcomers and*
*showing me the way to finally become one, too.*

*I love you both and admire you more than I ever*
*told you while you were here on earth. I could*
*not have hand-chosen better parents than you.*

# SWEET FREEDOM

x

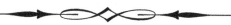

# AUTHOR'S NOTE

*"Fix your attention on God. You'll be changed from the inside out."*

Romans 12:2 MSG

8/20/21

M any are impressed when they learn I've lost over 260 pounds. To me, however, the more important thing is I've undergone a total lifestyle change of a slow, steady weight loss that lasts. I finally realized quick fixes do not work.

Once weighing 430 pounds, I've kept 250 pounds off for more than three years. To date, though, I've lost more than 260 pounds and am continuing to lose more.

In the past, my way of operating was to diet, lose weight and gain that weight back again, plus another 25 pounds or so. One step forward, three steps back. It was a frustrating way to live.

I've gone through a total metamorphosis, a transformation from the inside out.[1] It's a change which couldn't have happened unless I addressed the core issues holding me back. Today, I'm living in victory, and it's such a great feeling.

Overcoming emotional barriers has been a major key for me on my journey. In this process, God provided tools, truths and His leadership to heal emotions that held me back for years. In this book, I share how God used these in my life to show me the path to my own freedom.

With God's help I'm tearing down the barriers that had previously prevented me from keeping the weight off. Most of them are now behind me—a string as far as the eye can see. I'm sure some are ahead of me still. That's all right. I know how to cooperate with God for their removal.

## STRONGHOLDS

The barriers in my life caused me to run to food for comfort. I also allowed those same foods to become strongholds and take control of my life.

Those caught in different addictive cycles will also be able to see themselves in this book. My prayer is for anyone in any struggle to be able to identify the barriers and learn how to walk in freedom with God's help.

God set me free when I shut the door to the things that had become strongholds to me, the things I was allowing to take control of my life.

Strongholds are perpetuated by the evil one, the thief.[2] He wants me to run to food instead of God. In the end, it is always my choice. I can close the door on strongholds. This choice is only possible with God's help and only when I admit my weakness[3] to Him.

# WHO I AM

Many people ask, "Who are you and how are you qualified to write a book about weight loss?" It's simple. I'm just someone who has lost an extreme amount of weight, and have been able to keep it off. I also happen to be an author. I have a bachelor's degree in journalism and religion with a minor in psychology and a master's in Biblical studies. Writing is one of the giftings God gave me.

I am not a licensed professional counselor or an expert on healing emotions. However, I have become pretty good at listening to God, and following His leadership towards my total health. One thing I know for sure, if God hadn't led me to the tools I now use to confront my own emotional issues, I would still be on the gaining side again instead of the losing.

I am a spiritual coach, life purpose coach, writing coach, but most of all a Christian weight loss coach. As a former, super morbidly obese woman, I know what it is like to weight 430 pounds, and I know what it is like to lose 260 pounds. I've learned how to keep the weight off with God's help.

I'm fortunate to have been introduced to the Sozo ministry at Bethel Church and completed Bethel Sozo Beginning and Advanced Training.[4] Sozo is a Greek word meaning "saved, healed and delivered". To me the ministry is best described as a way to connect more deeply to God. It uses a combination of inner healing tools to help people do that.

I am a certified life purpose coach through Life Purpose Coaching Centers International®. This training was foundational in teaching me how to coach others in discovering the destiny God has for them.

As a coach, I utilize many tools I have learned through the years, as well as knowledge of how God led me to freedom. The stories in this book are my own experiences of how I walked out and am continuing to walk out my journey by overcoming barriers I created.

God is the best counselor. He can also use licensed professional counselors, physicians, nutitionists and trainers. I advise those with medical or emotional conditions to seek licensed professionals for additional assistance. I utilized all of these on my journey.

If you want to know how I won my battles while clinging tightly to Jesus, I tell you plainly in this book. I also have coaching groups and limited one-on-one coaching slots.

After all I've been through, God has now called me to share with others the path to freedom I have found. There are many ministries which utilize various inner healing techniques. I just happen to use them specifically with weight loss issues, and show with you how you can do it too.

## SWEET FREEDOM STUDY GUIDE

I developed *Sweet Freedom Study Guide* with the goal of helping you utilize many of the processes I refer to in this book. In the *Study Guide*, which can be purchased separately, I've included a section which describes the principles of inner healing which helped me, and the basics of how and why the tools work. The *Study Guide* also includes chapter-by-chapter Bible study, discussion questions and activities for your personal or group study. My goal was to make it as easy as possible for you to go on this journey.

In the introduction to *Sweet Freedom*, I share a synopsis of my journey. The first chapter discusses a foundational principle for utilizing the inner healing principles and for our lives. Any inner healing journey is designed to draw us closer to God. We can only do that when we know how to listen to Him and follow what He shows us. The rest of this book is my journey of physical, emotional and spiritual healing.

## STEPPING INTO FREEDOM

In 1994 at a Freedom Seminar, appropriately named, I joined with others declaring who they were. I made the prophetic proclamation that I was a whole, healthy, happy woman. At close to 430 pounds, I felt more like I was a broken, close-to-death, extremely sad blob.

More than two decades later, I can finally say I have stepped into that self-prophesy. I have learned my words are powerful. What I tell myself, as long as it aligns with God's desires for me, I will become.

If I were sitting across the table from you right now, I'd ask you, "Who are you? Who do you want to be?" That desire within you to become different than you currently are will profoundly direct you.

I wish you rich blessings as you travel with me deeper into the jungle of my journey. May this trip be as life-changing for you as it was for me.

Losing weight is good. Keeping it off is awesome. Being close to God, though, is truly where the sweetest of freedoms can be found.

## ENDNOTES

1.  Romans 12:2 MSG, AMP
2.  John 10:10 NIV
3.  2 Corinthians 12:9-10 MSG
4.  For more information go to http://bethelsozo.com.

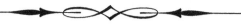

# C O N T E N T S

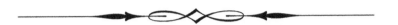

"*The Anointed One has set us free—not partially,
but completely and wonderfully free! We must
always cherish this truth and stubbornly refuse
to go back to the bondage of our past.*"

Galatians 5:1 TPT

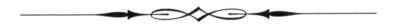

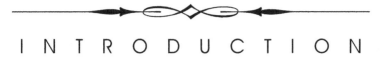

# INTRODUCTION

# BARRIERS

*"This means that anyone who belongs to Christ has become a new person. The old life is gone; a new life has begun!"*

2 Corinthians 5:17 NLT

One minute I was sitting in the green metal lawn chair in my uncle's front yard, talking and laughing with my aunt and cousins while the children played hide-and-go-seek.

The next minute, I felt the bending of the rounded legs as they slowly lowered me to the ground.

Even though I'm sure the sight of a 430-pound woman sitting atop a pile of metal was funny, all laughter stopped. My uncle jumped up to help me.

Being super morbidly obese I always tried to blend into the wallpaper and not make more of a spectacle of myself than I already was.

This day the proverbial cat had been let out of the bag. I was fat, really fat. I could break lawn chairs like twigs. I couldn't be trusted to sit anywhere.

My uncle brought me a sturdy dining room chair, which I eyed suspiciously. My aunt patted my arm and said, "It's fine. I never liked that old chair anyway." I wasn't fooled. I knew it was one of her favorites.

I was embarrassed for the rest of the day. I didn't dare eat the three to four platefuls I would have normally eaten at lunch. I took only one piece of cake, though I would have loved to have piled my plate with the four other desserts as well.

I knew I had a problem, even though I denied it constantly. I tried to push it under the rug. However, the day came when I could no longer ignore the obvious.

I felt I was a really good Christian. I didn't drink alcoholic beverages. I'd never done drugs, smoked cigarettes, had sex before marriage, gone to an X-rated movie, watched or listened to pornography. I went to church every Sunday. I taught Sunday School and small groups. I worked in ministry. And I was a glutton.

> The day came when I could no longer ignore the obvious...I was a glutton.

Any pastors I knew never talked about such things because they liked their sweets and breads as much as I did. I'd never heard gluttony called out from the pulpit, so I figured I didn't have to be concerned about it. Mine was the sanctified, unofficially church-approved sin.

It didn't matter until I began to break lawn chairs. Then the cardiac surgeon told me my body was too big for my heart and I would be dead in five years if I didn't lose a minimum of 100 pounds and keep it off.

Carrying hundreds of pounds of excess weight was like a living hell. It felt like I was putting on lead shirts every day. The burden got increasingly more intense, while I tried to be an increasingly more convincing actress.

"Yes, I'm fine. Everything is wonderful," was my answer to every off-handed, "How are you?"

I longed to say, "I'm drowning in a sea of my own making and I have no idea how to swim in this deep water." Instead, I learned to grin and bear it, even though the burden was unbearable and never one God meant for me to carry.

## LOSING WEIGHT AND KEEPING IT OFF

Almost anyone can lose weight, but most struggle and end up gaining it back again plus more. Losing weight is a challenge, but keeping it off is much harder. I've lost 100 pounds at least 10 or more times in my life. In the past it never stayed off because I always started eating the things I craved again

I could curtail what I ate for six months or so because I was looking forward to eating my favorite foods when I got to goal weight. The thought of the reward kept me good for limited periods of time.

I wanted to lose weight, but I just hadn't decided I needed to totally change my lifestyle. I wanted to lose the weight, but why did I start eating unhealthy foods again when I didn't want to gain it back and be a failure?

I knew gaining weight over and over again had to do with emotions in some way, but how could I ever discover the source of those deeply buried emotions and break their hold on me?

The key was not only finding them, but allowing God to help break the bonds. Losing weight is not painful, but cutting off the source of emotional ties, which caused the weight gain, can be.

Where did these tightly formed alliances come from? Many times we assume they come from the most recent problem or difficulty which started us eating again.

For instance, in 1980 I went on a diet and lost 100 pounds. The day I came back to lunch after weighing and finding out I had hit the magic mark, I got on the elevator to go my office. There was a department director on the elevator. I knew him by name only. I'd never had a conversation with him.

When the doors closed, he looked me up and down and said something like, "You're looking really good." Perhaps it was meant as a compliment, but the minute he spoke I froze, paralyzed with fear.

> Where did these tightly formed alliances come from?

By the time he said, "Let's talk sometime," my heart was pounding. Panic had set in. I was ready to run as soon as the elevator doors opened and I did.

That same day for afternoon break, I went down to the snack bar and bought several candy bars and a diet soda. At the time I didn't recognize my emotions were out of control. I calmed them the way I always had, with a sugary snack. I hadn't eaten candy bars in over a year. The day I lost the weight was the day I began putting it back on.

So what was the source of my weight gain? It was not the department director. He simply triggered a memory deep in my childhood. To deal with that issue, I had to identify the source. I had to go to the earliest time I felt that feeling. I needed to cut it off at the root by forgiving those involved, even if they meant no harm, and renouncing the lie God will treat me the same way the other person treated me. Then, I needed to hear His truth.

## PRESENTING ISSUES

Presenting issues are feelings which pop up at odd times. I found I must deal with these issues when they come up and not stuff them again with food like I had done most of my life. The moment God reveals the source is the moment of opportunity for healing.

The process is simple. It doesn't take much time if I am connected with God and prepared to listen when He wants to teach me. I recognize I have an issue and I take it to the Father in a time of prayer.

Sometimes He reveals the root of the issue in the moment and leads me in how to deal with it. Sometimes the insight comes later. I've dealt with issues sitting at a stoplight, driving down the highway, exercising, working, helping others through crises or smack dab in the middle of a church service. God gives me insights in an instant, which then sets me free in areas of deep wounding. I live for those moments of clarity.

Before I learned how to properly deal with these issues, my emotions were intrusive. They controlled me by making me cry, yell, stomp my feet or say mean things at inappropriate times. They could embarrass me if I allowed them to do so.

As a child I learned adults in my life didn't like these kinds of emotional outbursts. Truth be told, I didn't like myself when I felt the ugly emotions I didn't know how to handle. I discovered a quick and easy way to make them be quiet and not overwhelm me. I could just indulge, and even overindulge, in whatever food I craved. This would calm the emotions and they would be quiet for a while. It seemed to work well until it caused me to grow to life-threatening proportions.

## POWERING THROUGH

Upon reaching adulthood, I realized I had to lose weight. I didn't like being super morbidly obese. Plus, my size was greatly limiting my life. There would be times I had great resolve. I'd power through not listening to the emotions which told me to eat whatever I wanted.

Then, times of overwhelming stress, anger or loneliness would come and I would cave. I never thought I was an emotional eater because I didn't sit around crying and eating bonbons all day.

I did, however, celebrate with food. I would reward myself with food. I would comfort myself with food. I would protect myself with food. I would bolster my courage with food. Foods, especially those made with sugar and flour, were my go-to companions to deal with any crisis, large or small.

Going on a journey to freedom, I first had to go back and remember why I had allowed fears, lies, misconceptions, guilt, shame and so much more to become barriers in my life. Identifying the barriers, though, was a key to obtaining freedom. I had to have real faith that freedom would be mine some day. I had to have blind faith.

Faith is "the substance of things hoped for; the evidence of things not seen."[1] The Message says it this way, "The fundamental fact of existence is that this trust in God, this faith, is the firm foundation under everything that makes life worth living. It's our handle on what we can't see."[2]

I could only see myself at 430 pounds. I could not see myself as I am today, more than 260 pounds lighter. Yet, I had a hope in something I couldn't taste, touch, see, hear or smell.

The Amplified version says it best. "Now faith is the assurance, the confirmation, the title deed, of the things we hope for, being the proof of things we do not see and the conviction of their reality, faith perceiving as real fact what is not revealed to the senses."[3]

I like the concept of holding the title deed to what God promised me. If I hold the title deed to my home, it means it is mine. It is titled in my name. It will hold up in a court of law. To have the title deed to the faith I hope for means it is real. It has substance. I can count on it. It is fact, not wishful thinking.

## OBEDIENCE EQUALS FREEDOM

I never experienced the level of closeness I have today with Father God, Holy Spirit and Jesus. It comes from the truth that I love Him more than the things I used to love most in life—comfort foods.

When I stay close to God, He gives me the strength each day to say, "No," to the things I know will once again capture me if I let them. It's a simple choice. Do I want God or sugar? It really shouldn't even be a question I need to think about for an answer. My answer should automatically be God.

God's love blossomed in my life when I began to understand freedom costs me something. I surrendered everything to Him, even the foods I lived to eat. I began to allow Him to change me and make me new every day. It's not enough for me to be made new once. It's a process I must submit to each day to be renewed by the Holy Spirit.[4]

## SWEET FREEDOM

In this place of obedience, there is freedom, real freedom. It's not just flowery words. It is real, honest-to-goodness, I-feel-it-down-in the-tips-of-my-toes freedom.

When I go to a family gathering today, I am not pulled towards the desserts. I eat fruit, salad and meat. I make sure there are those choices because I bring them myself. Honestly, foods containing sugar and/or flour are not things I want, crave or desire to eat today. The longer I walk in obedience to what He has shown me to do, the more freedom I experience.

Sanctified sin does no one any good. It enslaves us the same as any other lifestyle contrary to God's best for us here on earth. It certainly never tastes as good as freedom feels.

I have learned many things on my journey, but probably the most important thing is how to listen, really listen, to God. Without hearing Him, listening to Him and following His instructions,[5] I would still be struggling with my weight, emotions and so much more.

## ENDNOTES

1. Hebrews 11:1 KJV
2. Hebrews 11:1 MSG
3. Hebrews 11:1 AMP
4. 2 Corinthians 5:17 AMP
5. John 10:27 NLT

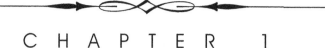

# C H A P T E R 1

# LISTEN

*"Come near to God and He will come near to you."*

James 4:8 NIV

---

Walking into my favorite grocery store when I was tired was not a good idea. I hadn't eaten that day and it was close to five. That morning I had solidified my decision and announced to my mentor that I would stop eating sugar and gluten. I would start cooking healthy. First I had to buy ingredients which would qualify. I needed to fix supper.

I had not thought about the looming obstacle I would encounter. I knew it was there. It's always there right as I head down the main aisle. That day it seemed to be larger and more intimidating than ever—the bakery case.

My downfall, the large cinnamon rolls, called to me. The voice in my head was urgent and loud. "You haven't eaten today. You need to eat something. You need energy. You might drop dead if you don't eat."

I listened to the voice and added my own rationalities. "I do have a long evening ahead, and I haven't eaten. I do need energy. I could grab these now and start the healthy eating thing tomorrow." I was telling myself this as I took a plastic bag, grabbed the tongs and had my two choice cinnamon rolls, the largest available, inside.

## GODS' VOICE

As I was tying the bag, I heard another voice in my head. This one was soft and quiet. It simply said, "What are you doing?"

The still, small voice arrested me. I had been on autopilot listening to the voice of the tempter who sided with my fleshly desires. All of sudden, I knew what I was preparing to do was everything I had vowed I would not do.

I put the bag back in the bakery case and went to choose my skinned and deboned chicken breasts, salad ingredients, broccoli and fruit. That was the last time I willingly listened to that overt voice.

## THE TEMPTER'S VOICE

For years, I listened to it all the time. The voice of the tempter always has an element of truth to it. What he tells me is half-truth, half-lie. In the past, he hadn't needed to be too subtle. He just put the bait out there and, like a hungry, naïve fish, I'd bite and gobble it up plus more. He would sit back with a smug smile while I swallowed the hook. His mission was accomplished.

Part of the reason I always listened to him was it sounded so logical. My rational mind agreed with him because my flesh wanted something sweet or starchy.

What the tempter didn't know was this time I was serious. I had made a firm decision. I was going to listen to the voice of God. I had invited Him to tell me when I was making a wrong decision.

## MY VOICE

I have learned my inner voice will mimic what is most important to me. In the past, I allowed my mind, my thoughts reasoning through things in my mind, to lead me. I thought this was the way my life was supposed to be run. My soul includes my mind, will and emotions, and I allowed my soul, of which my mind is a major part, to lead me.

I was a Christian. I considered myself to be spirit-led. However, my spirit was something nebulous to me. My spirit was weak because I wasn't allowing it to be led by God's Spirit. I had to put God's Spirit in charge of my spirit. My mind, will and emotions had to take a backseat.

There was a tug-of-war when I went in this direction. I had been allowing my mind to govern out of my soul's desires. So if my mind said, "You're hungry. Go ahead, eat that cinnamon roll or stop at that fast food drive-through," I would do it. My will agreed saying, "You can do whatever you want." My emotions kicked in as well telling me I deserved it. I needed comfort. I needed protection.

When I reserve something for myself, like my desire to eat whatever I want, whenever I want, then my voice will agree with the tempter. When I allow God's Spirit to lead me, my voice will agree with God. It's a choice. God always gives me a choice.

## HOW GOD SPEAKS

When I made the decision to eat healthy, I knew I couldn't do it on my own. By myself I am weak, but with God I am strong.[1] In my conversation with God, I said, "I can't do this without You. I've tried all my life to do it my way. Now I want to do it Your way. That means I submit to You completely in this area. Please remind me when I start to stray. Please guide me. Please give me the grace-power only You can provide."[2]

Because I had asked God to direct me, He did. He directed me through His voice speaking in my mind. It was different than the voice of evil. Instead of telling me to do something, God asked me to think about what I was doing.

God believed in me. He believed if I would use the brain He gave me, I would recognize the lie and go with the truth.

The grocery store instance, and many others throughout the years, taught me a lot about distinguishing the voices speaking in my head. I only want to listen to the voice of God. These days I can tell which voice is His.

## TOWARDS DESTINY

Starting to fulfill my destiny began with the Holy Spirit teaching me how to take care of my body. I couldn't go towards the purpose God had for my life when I was super morbidly obese and could barely walk. His desire was for me to become healthy so I could move to the next part of His plan for my life. The evil one knows this. He always hits at my weakness. As with everyone, my weakness is something born of a fleshly desire.

## TEN THINGS I'VE LEARNED ABOUT GOD'S VOICE

1. He will lead me to the whole truth,[3] not a half-truth.

2. He will not violate Scripture, but fulfill it.[4]

3. He will lead me towards my destiny, not away from it.[5]

4. He will redirect me according to His ultimate will.[6]

5. He will cause me to think rather than act on impulse.[7]

6. He will lead me away from fulfilling fleshly desires, and towards fulfilling my ultimate Kingdom purpose.[8]

7. He is loving, kind, understanding, soft and gentle.[9]

8. When I argue with Him, He doesn't argue back. He simply states a truth.[10]

9. He is always speaking to me, and speaks my language.[11]

10. I know His voice.[12]

For some it might be drugs, alcohol, sexual addiction, pornography, gambling, cigarettes, over-spending, or any number of things. These become things which pull God's children away from focusing on the main thing—God.

Jesus said it this way. "The thief comes only to steal, kill and destroy. I have come that they might have life and have it abundantly."[13] Satan's number one mission is to steal, kill and destroy my destiny. If he can, he will lead me off-course.

Every time the evil one did this, I had the nagging suspicion the voice speaking to me wasn't God. I listened, though, because it was something I wanted. After all, didn't God want me to be happy? This kind of thinking drove me to listen to the wrong voice.

## WHAT I WANT

My mind is not bad. When I became a Christian, I received the mind of Christ.[14] Learning to exercise it is another thing. I must be tuned in to God's station so my mind is functioning in conjunction with the Spirit of God. I must desire to be led by God rather than by my own desires.

When I want my way, I can have it because I have free will.[15] I can be just like Eve. My I-want voice can scream louder than the voice of God. The devil will agree with what I want. If I want to hear it, God's voice will whisper softly to me. That whisper will speak louder than every other voice combined if I let it.

I choose who I want to listen to. I really know the voice of God. I know what His purposes are. I know how to discern His voice. I just choose whether or not I want to follow it.

I don't know about you, but sometimes I doubt if it was God speaking to me or the junk food I ate last night. I can pretty much guarantee God was speaking while I was eating junk food.

The problem was not if God was speaking, it was am I listening with everything within me, with my heart, mind, and most of all, my spirit?

I base my interpretation of what I believe He is showing me on the truth of God's Word. Does it go contrary to Scripture? Is it Biblically based? Did my revelation come while I was meditating on His Word? If it did, I am always more encouraged it is God who is speaking to me.

When I get godly counsel, is it in agreement with what I believe I should do? This is not always an accurate test. I have to weigh the intentions of those advising me. Is their opinion based on time spent seeking God or just a whim?

Does it feel bigger than what I can accomplish? Lately, I've come to realize this is a part of what God is trying to teach me. If it's bigger than me, I will rely on Him. If not, I'll try to do it in my own strength. He leads me places I'm sure I can't go. If I will follow Him, instead of trying to lead the way, He will empower and protect me.

> God leads me places I'm sure I can't go. If I will follow Him, instead of trying to lead the way, He will empower and protect me.

"The LORD is my strength and my shield; my heart trusts in Him, and He helps me. My heart leaps for joy, and with my song I praise Him."[16]

My doubt is always removed when I read His promises. The words are life to me and tell me He's leading me into even greater things than I can ever imagine.

"Never doubt God's mighty power at work within you to accomplish all this. He will achieve infinitely more than your greatest request, your most unbelievable dream, and exceed your wildest imagination. He will outdo them all, for His miraculous power constantly energizes you."[17]

**He's got me. He won't let me go. No one can take me out of His hands.**

He's got me. He won't let go. No one can take me out of His hands.[18] The safest place for me is following His voice, attempting the impossible with Him.[19]

Jesus said, "My sheep hear My voice, and I know them, and they follow Me."[20] Why do sheep follow the voice of the shepherd? Because they trust him. He protects them. He feeds them. He finds water for them, shelter when needed and soft places to lie down.

When I began to understand God wanted only good things for me, not disaster,[21] I began to listen to His advice. I longed for His voice.

I began to live my life based on what He said to me. I began to hear Him everywhere. His is a voice which fills all of me. There is no other voice like it.

"Then he (Elijah) was told, 'Go, stand on the mountain at attention before God. God will pass by.' A hurricane wind ripped through the mountains and shattered the rocks before God, but God wasn't to be found in the wind; after the wind an earthquake, but God wasn't in the earthquake; and after the earthquake fire, but God wasn't in the fire; and after the fire a gentle and quiet whisper.

"When Elijah heard the quiet voice, he muffled his face with his great cloak, went to the mouth of the cave, and stood there. A quiet voice asked, 'So Elijah, now tell Me, what are you doing here?'"[22]

The voice of God doesn't have to be a "voice" at all. It can be His presence. It can be a look on stranger's face. It can be warm sunshine on my back. It can be a boisterous seven-year-old giving a hug to one of his best friends. It can be a three-year-old crawling up in her grandmother's lap. It can be a friend giving an unsolicited hug. Or it can be a sense of purpose and a knowing that I just can't get out of my mind.

## WAS IT AN AUDIBLE VOICE?

In 1979 when a pastor of a large church announced he was not running for a second term as president of one the largest denominations in the world, people were stunned. He said he was not running because God told him not to.

A reporter asked him, "Did God speak to you in an audible voice?" The pastor looked him in the eyes and said, "No, it was much louder than that."[23]

I know God directs me when I'm willing to listen. He has hope for me no matter what predicament I've gotten myself into. Hope in God and His strength is my lifeline, the steadfast and sure anchor of my very being.[24]

For years, I had a hard time learning how to overcome my feeling of being hopelessly overweight. Where did it begin?

## ENDNOTES

1.  2 Corinthians 12:10 NIV

2.  2 Corinthians 12:9 MSG

3.  John 14:6 NIV

4.  Numbers 23:19 NIV

5.  Jeremiah 29:11 NLT

6.  Isaiah 30:21 NLT

7.  Ephesians 5:15-17 NIV

8.  Galatians 5:16-18 NIV

9.  James 3:17 NIV

10. Psalm 25:5 NIV

11. Jeremiah 33:3 NIV

12. John 10:27 NLT

13. John 10:10 NASB

14. 1 Corinthians 2:16 NIV

15. Genesis 2:16-17, 3:6 NIV

16. Psalm 28:7 NLT

17. Ephesians 2:20 TPT

18. John 10:29 NIV

19. Luke 1:37 NIV

20. John 10:27 ESV

21. Jeremiah 29:11 NLT

22. 1 Kings 19:11-13 MSG

23. Wilkins, Tim. "Hearing God's Voice. An Auditory Art?" Hearing God's Voice. An Auditory Art? Cross Ministry.org, n.d. Web. 26 Dec. 2015.

24. Hebrews 6:19 NIV

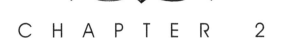

C H A P T E R 2

# HOPELESS

*"My grace is enough. It's all you need. My power
comes into its own in your weakness."*

2 Corinthians 12:9 MSG

---

can't lose weight, I just can't. I had carried this feeling of defeat with me for as long as I can remember. Growing up, I was always outgrowing my clothes. Hey, it's what kids do. They grow.

When I look at my pictures from when I was grade school age, it seems I grew faster than other kids. There is an old picture of me holding my little sister on my hip. She was still a baby, probably eight months old. I would have been almost nine. However, I was nearly as tall and as large as my grandmother. At nine I was the size of an adult woman.

I can remember being several sizes larger than those in my classes. I always felt fat compared to the smaller, popular girls. I just seemed to grow faster than others my age. My growth spurts caused a bit of angst on the family budget, which my mother monitored carefully. "We don't have money to keep buying you new clothes every time we turn around," she'd say. "You're growing too fast."

I remember statements like this when I outgrew anything—shoes, coats, jeans, dresses. I was the oldest. There was no one to hand things down to me. Everything had to be bought new.

## STOP GROWING

I wished I could stop growing, be smaller, petite and pretty like the girls in my class. I began puberty at age nine, which meant I needed different underwear in addition to other clothes. Everything about me was changing, and I hated it because I felt like a huge inconvenience to my family.

Sometimes I would think about not eating. Then, I'd feign sickness, but in a few hours I would be back saying I was hungry. I felt like a failure. I knew I was doomed to continue to gain weight. It was just some weird quirk within me. I was fat and always would be.

My mother would say, "You'll eat us out of house and home." I was hopeless.

One day I overheard Mom and Grandma talking about what clothes I needed. It was the middle of the school year and normally we didn't buy clothes except at the beginning of school.

Mom said, "She just keeps gaining weight. She's in husky sizes. I can't find anything in girls' sizes to fit her and women's sizes don't fit her yet. If they fit in the waist, they are way too big in the top. She's got to stop gaining weight, but it's like she just can't stop eating." Mom's voice was a loud, frustrated whisper. I knew her statements were not ones she meant for me to hear.

Grandma said, "It's nothing to fret about. She can't help it. Kids have to eat. God gave her a healthy appetite. She's a good kid."

Even Grandma said I couldn't help gaining weight, and Mom said I can't stop eating. I just allowed what I perceived as truth to sink in and take root. What else can a kid do when the two maternal figures in her life agree? It felt entirely like a truth.

"I can't lose weight. I'm hopeless," I told myself over and over.

## HALF-TRUTH

It was true, as a child I couldn't lose weight. I was designed to grow, not lose weight. The difficult part, especially for a child, is separating out what is true and what is a lie. A child is not meant to understand all of this. They are to be loved and supported by the adults in their lives. They are not supposed to overhear conversations which make them feel like they are helpless and hopeless.

Scripture says it this way, "When I was a child, I talked like a child, I thought like a child, I reasoned like a child; when I became a man (or woman), I did away with childish things."[1]

I did not have the capacity to think or reason through what was true and what was false. In most cases, children can go to their parents to learn the truth. My mother had an emotional illness, and I didn't think I could ask her what she meant. I didn't want to ask my grandmother or my father because if they agreed with her, I was doomed.

## I BELIEVED A LIE

I believed my mother. I had evidence to support what she said. I was growing, gaining weight, needing larger size clothes. I was larger than every girl in my class. It became a core belief. I can't lose weight, except this was a lie.

In high school, I was in marching band for one semester. An hour of early morning band practices three days a week for about three months at the beginning of my sophomore year netted a 20-pound weight loss. It should have showed me I could lose weight if I exercised. Instead, I was just frustrated with having to get to school by seven in the morning.

Of course, when band season ended I put the weight right back on, especially with Thanksgiving, Christmas, New Year's Eve and Grandma's, Mom's, Papaw's, Dad's, aunts, uncles and cousins birthdays falling in line. Every month there was a holiday or birthday to celebrate. Our family went all out for every such occasion. Food, food and more food marked each special event. It's who we were. It's how I grew up. It further reinforced the idea—I can't lose weight.

I accepted the call to be a missionary when I was in junior high during a service when a missionary showed slides of brown-eyed Latin American children. Several years later I wound up working in the press office of the Foreign Missions Board. It was as close as I could get to the mission field without a seminary degree. While there, I applied to a two-year mission program for college graduates. I was excited about serving overseas. Imagine my deflated ego when I got the letter saying I was rejected unless I lost 30 pounds in 10 weeks, the starting date of the program.

My desire for embarking on a career as a missionary ended right there. I didn't even try to lose weight. By age 21, I had fully accepted the embedded lie that I couldn't lose weight. It was an impossibility.

I was sure my reactions to situations, especially situations involving food, were just my personality. It was just who I was and how I responded. I accepted these lies as facts.

I know now there are many lies I perceived as truth and began believing as a child. For some reason, I wasn't able to sort these out when I became an adult. I knew the lies were attached to the way I viewed food, but I had no idea where to start to figure it all out.

## IDENTIFYING LIES

The only place I could begin was the place where truth is found. Of course, real truth is present only in God's Word. First, I had to try to dig through the tons of emotional garbage to find where the lies were hiding.

Identifying lies can be an exhausting and even impossible process. When my mind would begin to figure something out and connect the dots, confusion would set in. My brain would worry the ideas and concepts to death until I was exhausted.

It wasn't until I allowed myself to go to the deep places that I began to uncover the core falsehoods which were guiding my life. I had no idea of the depth of these lies, nor of the truths the enemy was trying to keep me from understanding.

## WHAT IS THE TRUTH?

In order for God to get my attention with His truth on this subject, He needed to show me how untrue the statement, "I can't lose weight," was. To do that, He had to jolt me into the reality of my predicament.

In 1999 I was in the hospital for a possible mitral valve replacement. I weighed 430 pounds. I vividly remember the cardiac surgeon walking into my room and telling me, "You don't need heart surgery. You need to lose weight. Your heart was never designed to pump blood through a body of your size. You need to lose 100 pounds and keep it off or you will be dead in five years."

So, I lost 100 pounds by going on a high protein diet. Like all the other times, though, I began gaining the weight back after losing it. I kept it off longer, but I began eating sugar again. Every time I began eating sugar, I would gain weight again. I'd put the weight back on plus more.

The truth I discovered is I can't maintain weight loss if I eat sugar. When I start eating sugar, I can't stop. For me, it's extremely addictive.

To clarify, by sugar I mean all foods which quickly convert to large amounts of sugar in the bloodstream. Growing up my mother called these "starches". This includes white bread, hot rolls, quick breads, pastas, noodles, spaghetti, macaroni, potatoes, corn, rice, chips and snacks, doughnuts, cakes, cookies, cereals and all things made with flour or wheat.

Like a nurse practitioner I know says, "Eating a mound of mashed potatoes is like eating a mound of sugar." It is a food with a high glycemic index, which means it quickly raises the blood glucose or sugar level in the blood. When I eat a food with a high glycemic index my body gets a sugar high followed quickly by a crash. Then, I want more of that same substance to get the same feeling.

It is very addictive because now I need a greater quantity to get the same rush. This begins the craving cycle. It's why I used to think I couldn't live without sugar and breads.

"I can't lose weight" was a truth for me because most everything I ate had some element of starchy foods. Sure, I ate meats, fruits and vegetables. Meats were breaded and fried. Vegetables were covered in a rich starchy sauce and fruits were in pies.

> Alcohol is one molecule away from sugar. Alcohol is liquid sugar.

For many years I wallowed in this place of "I can't lose weight". Rooted in my childhood, this belief went deep into me, and stayed until God brought me face-to-face with reality.

I was in a meeting. My mentor, a long-time sober alcoholic, was telling his story. I was only halfway listening. This doesn't relate to me, I thought. I settled the alcohol thing a long time ago. All of a sudden, though, his words captivated me.

"Alcohol is one molecule away from sugar. Alcohol is liquid sugar."

Like a magnet, the pieces of my life snapped together. I can't lose weight because I am a sugar addict. This was before all the hub-bub about sugar addiction. I'd not heard anything about it. I didn't even know if it was a real "thing." I just knew as I looked back over my life, the reason I was held captive in my body was because I couldn't not eat sugar. I had never realized how paralyzed I was by the substance. I was weak around it. I wanted it constantly.

All my life I had wished my problem was alcohol instead of food. My reasoning was an alcoholic could stop drinking alcohol because it is not necessary for survival.

I can't stop eating, however, because I have to eat to survive. I wasn't eating to survive, though. I was living to eat, as much as I wanted, any time I wanted.

Understanding sugar, flour and starches are my nemeses gave me the final motivation to do what God had been telling me to do for more than 30 years.

## GOD'S PLAN

In 1977, I was reading my morning devotional when a familiar passage popped up. "'You don't have enough faith,' Jesus told them. 'I tell you the truth, if you had faith even as small as a mustard seed, you could say to this mountain, 'Move from here to there,' and it would move. Nothing would be impossible.'"[2]

I had been gaining more weight, at least 50 pounds since I had gotten married. I felt like a mountain. He said if I have faith the mountain will move. So, I cried out and asked Him, "How can I move this mountain of flesh?" I was surprised at His quick answer. He gave me a plan. I wrote it in my prayer journal. "Stop eating sugar. Eat more meats, fruits and vegetables, and stop eating so much bread."

## MY PLAN

I also wrote my response. "Nice plan, God. I'd lose weight if I did that, but I can't stop eating sugar. There's no way. Let me try it my way." For the next 30 years I tried to have my cake (weight loss) and eat it, too (the literal cake). This plan, no matter how I ordered it, did not work.

My plan would work until I lost down to a goal weight. Then, I'd reward myself with some sugary treat. See, I reasoned God surely didn't mean stop eating sugar altogether. Everyone deserves a little sugar now and then, don't they?

The problem was, I could never stop with just a little. The look, the smell, the taste of something enormously sweet would set up what I perceived as a need for more and more and more.

So I asked my mentor, "Is it possible to be addicted to sugar?"

"You can be addicted to anything which controls you," he answered.

Immediately my stomach fell to the floor. I am a sugar addict. The truth of it was something I instantly knew. In that moment, my life shifted.


## MORBID OBESITY IS NOT SUPER

I had gone through weight loss surgery and had lost weight. The reality I didn't want to face was I had already started my trend of gaining weight back. I was headed back to super morbid obesity and beyond. I didn't want to die, but I knew I was severely limiting any quality time I had on earth.

Super morbid obesity is not a place most people intentionally want to go. When I was there, though, it seemed some normal weight people thought I was gaining weight on purpose because they had no problem maintaining a healthy weight. I know it's difficult for others to understand because it was difficult for me to understand.

I hated hurting every time I took a step. I hated not being able to walk through the large discount stores without sitting down every two aisles. I hated not being able to buy clothes anywhere, except from a catalog or online. I hated not being able to go on amusement rides with my kids or walk around a park or zoo.

I hated not being able to fit in chairs, booths, cars, pews, amusement rides, airplane seats and train seats. I hated having no energy. I hated being a burden to my family. I hated the way I looked. I hated the way I felt. I hated myself.

I know the literal hell of it. I have been there. I never want to go back. Yet, I was on a bullet train right back there. I also knew I had tried everything imaginable to lose weight and keep it off. Everything, that is, but God's plan. He gave me the same plan many times throughout my life. I have it recorded in my journal. In addition to 1977, there was 1982, 1986, 1990, 1998 and maybe a few I missed.

**I hated the way I looked. I hated the way I felt. I hated myself.**

The message was consistent. The answer was there in front of me all the time. It was evident in the way I could lose weight and regain it so quickly. Why had I never accepted it before?

I had allowed an emotion to become a core life value. The only way I can describe it is hopelessness. My mother and my grandmother's words left me feeling hopeless. I accepted them as facts. I can't lose weight. I'll never be able to lose weight. All I do is gain weight.

When the emotion of hopelessness over my situation would surface there would be only one recourse for me. I would eat, preferably something made with sugar and flour, something like my grandmother would have made.

I fed the hopelessness inside me with the only thing I knew would quiet it. This allowed me to go about with a somewhat normal state of emotions. It would anesthetize my pain for a short while. Then, I'd need more to get the same feeling. If this sounds like an addictive cycle, it is.

> When I finally came to the end of myself and totally surrendered to what God had been telling me, my life transformed completely.

I continued to do this through various trials and temptations, always giving in, never taking a stand. When I finally came to the end of myself and totally surrendered to what God had been telling me, my life transformed completely.

The switch in my brain happened quickly, the second I recognized the truth. The truth is I can lose weight if I stop eating sugar. The reality of how to do this was the challenge. I was, and still am, like Paul. I have a weakness. Scripture doesn't tell us what Paul's weakness was. It does tell us he asked God three times to remove it.

Eventually he realized, "So I wouldn't get a big head, I was given the gift of a handicap to keep me in constant touch with my limitations. Satan's angel did his best to get me down; what he in fact did was push me to my knees. No danger then of walking around high and mighty! At first I didn't think of it as a gift, and begged God to remove it. Three times I did that, and then he told me, 'My grace is enough; it's all you need. My strength comes into its own in your weakness.'"[3]

> There were times I was sure my issue was so big even God couldn't help me.

Paul learned humanity has limitations. Those limitations, though, are not reasons to quit. They should lead me to understand, the weaker I am, the stronger I can become when I rely totally on God's strength instead of my own.[4]

My weakness for certain foods was there to help me understand I need to rely more fully on God. Instead, I took things into my own hands and made the mess bigger and bigger until I got to the point I knew beyond a shadow of a doubt, I couldn't overcome the pull certain foods have on me without God's help.

Yet, there were times I was sure my issue was so big even God couldn't help me. My lifeline was what God told Paul. "My grace is enough. It's all you need. My strength comes into its own in your weakness."[5]

Sometimes Scripture has a gentle way of showing me truth, and sometimes it hits me in the gut with such force, I know I will never forget its truth. Why could I never before access God's power? I would pray. I would cry out for help. Every time He'd give me the same answer about stopping sugar, and every time I would say I can't do it. Why didn't He just zap me with His power, fix me, make everything right or send down a lightning bolt?

As long as I was trying to do it on my own, I had rendered His power useless in my life. Is God strong all the time? Yes, He is. Why was His strength not activated in my life? His power is only made complete when I admit my weakness and abject poverty in this area.

I said I needed help. In reality, the help I wanted was to keep doing what I was doing, eating what I wanted to eat, but get different results. This is the definition of insanity. I fully admit I was there. I was insane to think I could do the same thing and get different results.

> I wanted to keep doing what I was doing, eating what I wanted to eat, but get different results.

The first step in any radical change is to do something different. I wanted to keep everything the same, but lose weight. I had a lot of passion about losing weight. I knew all the reasons why I should lose weight. I knew the practicality behind it. I'd be eager to go on a diet. For the first day, I would have great resolve. Then, somewhere along the way, I would fail.

"What I don't understand about myself is that I decide one way, but then I act another, doing things I absolutely despise … I can will it, but I can't do it. I decide to do good, but I don't really do it; I decide not to do bad, but then I do it anyway. My decisions, such as they are, don't result in actions. Something has gone wrong deep within me and gets the better of me every time."[6]

"I've tried everything and nothing helps. I'm at the end of my rope. Is there no one who can do anything for me? Isn't that the real question?"[7]

This is exactly how I felt. I knew the truth from what God had told me throughout the years, all the times I had cried out to Him and He gave me the same answer. I couldn't act like I didn't know. I was going to have to let go of my best friend, sugar.

## SURRENDER

This felt a whole lot like surrender and I don't mean in a good way. I mean surrender as in being captured by the enemy. However, I was already captured by the enemy. What God had been telling me for years was surrendering to Him is the only way to freedom. How I had gotten it so backwards is beyond me.

The key is in the next verse, but it had always eluded me. "The answer, thank God, is that Jesus Christ can and does. He acted to set things right in this life of contradictions where I want to serve God with all my heart and mind, but am pulled by the influence of sin to do something totally different."[8]

Then, I saw it clearly. I had been looking in the wrong place. Acting in my own human strength, I will always be waffling. If I really understand the grace of God, I will understand His strength can't operate when I'm acting self-sufficient, self-important, holier than even God.

This is when God says, "OK, I'll wait until you really know you need and want Me." When I'm at the end of my rope, when I've truly exhausted every resource and when it hits me hard enough for me to know all of this, God says, "Now you're ready. Let's go."

**I pushed start on God's power button for my life.**

Any weakness I have is only meant to draw me closer to God. He knows I am weak. It's why He gives me grace.[9] When I surrendered my wants and desires, I pushed start on God's power button for my life.

It's all based in grace. It's grace-power. It's always available until I take matters back into my own hands and stop listening to His direction. When this happens, I pull the plug on the God-power generator and I do things in my strength.

There can only be one power source at a time. I must choose—my way or God's way.

When I began to walk out what I knew was His plan, I felt His grace-wind at my back propelling me forward to health and wholeness. It's a place from which I can minister. It's a place from which I can complete my assignment here on earth. It's a place from which I can live.

There would be more, so much more I would learn on my journey, especially about my obsessive need to control everything and everyone. Why did I feel I had to do it or it wouldn't get done? Wasn't that a good trait to have?

The roots of control traced back to what seemed an unlikely root. I was about to find the evil one loves to hide roots in places we wouldn't think of looking.

ENDNOTES

1. 1 Corinthians 13:11 AMP
2. Matthew 17:20 NLT
3. 2 Corinthians 12: 7-9 MSG
4. 2 Corinthians 12:10 MSG
5. 2 Corinthians 12:9 MSG
6. Romans 7: 15, 18-20 MSG
7. Romans 7:24 MSG
8. Romans 7:25 MSG
9. Ephesians 2:8-9 TPT

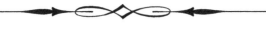

CHAPTER 3

# CONTROL

*"God elevated Him to the place of highest honor and gave Him the name above all other names, that at the name of Jesus every knee should bow, in heaven and on earth and under the earth, and every tongue declare that Jesus Christ is Lord, to the glory of God the Father."*

Philippians 2:9-11 NLT

A s the oldest grandchild on my mother's side of the family, I was center-stage and I knew it. There are tons of pictures of me, and it is apparent I was doted on by my parents and grandparents.

I was two and a half years old when my little brother was born. I was sharing the stage with a sibling for the first time. One of the first stories I remember my mother telling about the new baby gives me a clue as to how I felt about having a baby brother.

My grandmother had brought him an outfit to come home from the hospital. It included a pair of baby booties made to look like little shoes. Everyone was raving about how grown-up Randy looked in his new little shoes. I guess I'd had quite enough of the attention my baby brother was getting.

Maybe what I said was a foreshadowing of what kind of big sister I would be. "Well, put him down and let him walk then."

It's crazy, but I can remember how I felt—arms crossed, toe tapping with a frown on my face. Everyone was laughing and paying more attention to my new baby brother than to me.

I was supposed to love him immensely, instead I was immediately jealous. Someone else was stealing the limelight. I know this is not unusual. It is how most oldest siblings feel when a new baby joins the family, but I had to learn life is not about me.

## IMPOSSIBLE NOT TO LOVE

My little brother was impossible not to love. One thing which endeared him to me was that until he was about four years old, I was the only one who could understand what he was saying. So, I became his interpreter.

Many times my mother would get exasperated because she couldn't understand him. I'd tell her what he said. He'd shake his head yes indicating I had correctly interpreted, and I would feel needed and appreciated once again

Perhaps it was my need to be noticed, but I distinctly remember feeling I had contributed something valuable to my family. After that, I more easily slipped into the role of big sister. I decided if I couldn't be the center of attention, I could be helpful. I had no idea what I was setting myself up for later.

My mother's emotional illness began to get worse through the years. By 1959, she was having episodes of anxiety and depression.

When I asked Grandma about it, she said, "Your mother has always been frail." Dad's answer was, "She's sick." Later my aunt would say she felt my mother's illness started when a baby daughter was stillborn when I was 15 months old. Whatever the reason, it had been present in her life for a long time. It certainly seemed to have been there for as long as I could remember.

As a child full of questions, these answers did not satisfy me, but it was all I was told. What I did know was my mother needed help around the house. I can't remember a time when I didn't do chores.

By the time I was seven, I could make a basic meal of hot dogs, fish sticks, hamburgers or chili. Microwaves didn't exist back then, so I had to use the stove. I could also mix up and bake a batch of cookies, butterscotch brownies or a cake.

> She could be angry and upset, but pick up a book, get lost in the story and be calm and enraptured for hours.

I knew how to use the washer and dryer. I could clean our small five-room house in an hour. I was also making sure I knew where my brother was at all times.

In other words, I was running the household. At this point, my mother was functional, but she was withdrawing more and more. Most of the time, her withdrawal would be into a fictional book. She read books voraciously.

She could be angry and upset, but pick up a book, get lost in the story and be calm and enraptured for hours. It made me think of when David played the harp for Saul.[1] Whatever was harassing her would leave for just a span of time. When I saw books calm her my desire to become an author began.

I was eight when my baby sister was born. She was a beautiful, blonde-haired bundle of joy. I loved her, and I claimed her as my own immediately. I loved to take care of her, give her a bath, change her diaper and get her dressed.

There were now three children in a tiny house. More noise, more mouths to feed, more clothes to buy all added to my mother's continual emotional downward spiral. She had an emotional illness. It didn't go away even with continual visits to psychiatrists and taking different high-powered medications.

> More noise, more mouths to feed, more clothes to buy all added to my mother's continual emotional downward spiral.

What it all meant for me was I took over most of her duties. She got to the point where she would not go out of the house.

Dad worked, but would be home right after work. He didn't cook or clean. He did errands such as getting the meat from the locker and going to the grocery store. I went with him to help because he had no idea what to purchase.

I managed the house, did housework, laundry, cooked supper, took care of the kids and did my own homework and school activities. I was concerned about my mother, but I did not really understand what her "sickness" entailed. I was glad to help where I could.

The summer I was 12, my mother went into the hospital for several months. I had total responsibility for my siblings during that time. I felt overwhelmed. There was so much I didn't know how to do. I was inadequate a lot of the time, still I wanted to help.

**The desire to help quickly became overshadowed by the fear of failure.**

I would burn the chili or put in cinnamon instead of chili powder. I juggled taking care of my little sister, while cooking supper and keeping an eye on my brother. The desire to help quickly became overshadowed by the fear of failure. I improvised a lot, and somehow, I'm sure only by God's grace, I got it done and my brother and sister survived intact.

I never blamed anyone for this time period in my life. After all, Mom was "sick", Dad had to work and Grandma was 30 miles away, which seemed a huge distance back then. I was even forbidden to call her because long distance charges were expensive.

I felt alone and trapped without a plan or resources. However, it made me a better person, stronger and able to handle or face anything. I became the bossy, oldest child. It was a works mentality, and I fell into it naturally, so much so I thought it was just who I was supposed to be. I'm the responsible child. I'm the one who gets everything done. Someone has to do it.

It was several years ago that I began studying about types of emotional healing. I learned the things I perceive as a child in regard to my biological family affect how I feel about God.

This approach appealed to me because I knew I had healing to do in regard to my relationship with my mother.

My siblings and I have always been close. However, in the emotional healing process I was studying how my relationship with my siblings can affect my relationship with Jesus. I knew I should check to see if everything was solid.

One of the first steps in the process was to picture who Jesus is to me. Not who I think He should be, but who I feel He is. This helps tap into the emotions which can override any knowledge, even Scriptural knowledge, I have of Jesus.

## THE JESUS PICTURE

I had done this many times. The picture which always came to mind was one I painted of Jesus many years ago. It hangs on my living room wall. Jesus is smiling and laughing and dressed in a muslin and burlap robe. It speaks of the Jesus who walks and travels this journey with me. I've always felt it is a perfect depiction of my Jesus.

When I began to picture who Jesus is to me, this painting automatically came to my mind. I was about to move on, when something about the picture made me gasp. It was exactly the same picture. It hadn't changed. That was the problem. It was a two-dimensional, flat painting, a static object. It was not three-dimensional. It was not alive. It was not a real person. It was not the real Jesus.

I asked, "Jesus, what lie am I believing about You?" Immediately, I saw a motion picture moving through my memory. It was of my brother, my sister and some neighbor kids laughing and playing tag in the back yard. Jesus was one of the kids, running and playing.

I was the big sister standing on the back patio, hands on my hips, telling them it was too late to be playing outside. All of the kids, including Jesus, begged me for just a few more minutes.

"Please let us play," Jesus said. "We are having fun. It's not dark yet and look, the neighbors are still sitting out. Can't we have a little longer, please? Can't we?"

And the picture froze.

"Oh, Jesus," I mourned. "I think I'm bigger than You. I think I can tell You what to do."

Some revelations are glorious and some hit you in the middle of your gut so hard you think you are going to be sick. This was the latter.

**It was such a big lie that I had not seen it.**

I clearly saw I was jealous of my brother and sister being able to just be carefree kids, playing and having fun while I was working. I was jealous because even though I didn't want to play, I felt resentment because I didn't feel free to do so.

I felt validation for being needed to do the adult work, but I saw clearly I also wanted to be a kid. It was twisted in my mind so much it was hard for me to delineate. The bottom line was I felt Jesus was not being responsible and I was. I had to take care of the situation because no one else would.

It was such a big lie that I had not seen it. It was bigger than my view of the situation. All these years, it was hiding behind the smiling painting of Jesus. I understood immediately it had to do with my works mentality. I had never been able to get to the cause of that because I had been looking in the wrong place.

I understood how looking in the wrong place is possible. I was reminded of a woman I was leading through an inner healing session. When she came into the room, I sensed she was fearful. Many times God will show me something like this. Usually it means it's a good place to start the inner healing process.

## DOOR OF FEAR

I asked her to go to the door of fear in her mind and tell me if it was open or closed. Open would usually mean fear has invaded her life. Closed usually means there is no fear. She said it was closed. I asked her to examine it carefully to see if there was any crack or ability for the door to come open. She said, "No, it is closed solidly."

This was baffling to me because I still sensed great fear. We moved on and dealt with a few other things which are usually fear-related. For instance, how we view God the Father ,which relates to our view of our earthly father who is our protector. Everything was fine there.

I said, "There are a few more doors we can investigate, shall we go there?" We went to the door of hatred, then sexual sins. We dealt with different things in each door, but we still had not found the fear.

"There is one more door. Shall we try it?"

"What is it?" she asked.

44

"The door of witchcraft. I've never dealt with anyone who had anything there, but I think we should try it just to see."

She felt she had nothing there, but agreed. She remembered an incident in her childhood when she was at a sleep over and they played with a Ouija board. She had been told never to do that. As a child she was scared of even trying. When she did, the board seemed to move and spell out a name.

The name belonged to someone of whom she was afraid when she was a child. She had buried the memory associated with the person because she was afraid even God could not deal with the revelation.

She was surprised to discover these feelings. The very unveiling of it brought fear. Slowly we went through the process of handing the person and the fear to Father God. In exchange, God gave her peace and the weapons of warfare.

She was visibly moved when she handed the person to God. I asked her, "What just happened?"

She said, "A dark cloud I've been living under all my life has lifted. I think I'm able to trust God now." Her fear and trust issues were hiding behind a different door. They had been buried deep because the little girl version of herself did not know how to handle them.

## HIDDEN ISSUES

I sensed this same thing was happening with me. My training in inner healing told me it would be natural for a father or father figure to be the source of my disposition towards works, self-effort and striving to earn Father God's favor, but I knew the source was not there.

My works mentality was not found in the aspect of my dad, who worked hard at his job and ministry. He did both out of love for his family and for God.

It was hiding in a most unlikely place—my siblings. Hidden lies, the ones I can't reason through, are some of the hardest lies to uncover, but also lead to the greatest revelations. Sometimes they are hidden because the things I need to forgive are not wrong actions on the others' parts. They are simply wrong perceptions on my part.

## FORGIVING MY SIBLINGS

To get free, I must go through forgiveness to set free the emotions of the child, which still exist within me. These emotions govern most of my actions and behaviors, especially the ones I try to stop. They are the reason I can't seem to change my habits and feelings no matter how hard I try. They will override my rational thinking every time unless I get to the root of why they are hanging around.

I prayed, "I forgive my brother and sister for being kids, for playing and for having fun while I could not bring myself to enter in. I forgive them for their carefree attitudes and their overall enjoyment of life. I forgive them for being needy and for me feeling like I had to take care of them. I forgive myself for feeling better or bigger or more important than them. I forgive myself for never enjoying life."

The important part of the process is to renounce the lies this brings up about Jesus. I do this because my siblings, like Jesus, are the ones who are most like me. Among the Godhead, Jesus was the one who walked on earth. He knows what it's like to be human. My siblings are my earliest companions. They lived with me and we have many of the same life experiences.

This part was extremely difficult for me to pray and even harder to admit. I had been carrying these deeply buried lies for years. I was tired of laboring under the burden. I was ready to be free.

"I renounce the lie that You, Jesus, are my younger brother who just plays all the time and doesn't take anything serious. I renounce the lie You are carefree while requiring me to work all the time and not play or enjoy life. I renounce the lie You prefer me not to enjoy life. I renounce the lie that I am bigger than You."

I wept knowing the depth of the lie I was admitting.

Drying my tears, I asked, "Jesus, what is Your truth?" His response was immediate, like a voice booming from above. It made me want to stand at attention. It was not audible, but I felt the power of it all the same.

> I had been carrying these deeply buried lies for years. I was tried of laboring under the burden.

"Teresa, I am Jehovah Jirah (the Lord will provide), Jehovah Rapha (the Lord who Heals), Jehovah Shammah (The Lord is There), Jehovah-Tsidkenus (the Lord our Righteousness). I am the all powerful One. There is none greater than Me.[2] I am your Creator. I am your Redeemer. I am your Savior. I am all you need. Hand Me your wrong thinking, your wrong beliefs, and I will hand you the real picture."

The following moments were powerful. I saw a loving, smiling Jesus with strong muscular arms and large hands. He sat down and entreated me to come to Him. He held me close and told me He would never leave me. He told me I was important to Him.

He said, "Rest with me. Nothing is required of you except staying close to Me." In that place, time stood still. He was right. Nothing else mattered.

## EMOTIONS—DEAD OR ALIVE?

No matter what I think, there are many areas I have decided won't harm me and so I have buried the emotions attached to them. I think I have buried these and they are dead. Instead I found I buried many of my emotions alive. They would scream and shout at me. I would try to keep them quiet by hiding them under hundreds of pound of fat and tons of emotional baggage.

Many of these emotions have held me back in some way on my weight loss journey. Jesus is the member of the Godhead who lived as a human here on earth. He completely understands the hazards I have and will encounter while traveling this journey. I need Him as my mentor to walk with me.

With Him I can do all things.[3] Without Him, I am toast. I cannot deal with any overriding life issues, addictions, difficult relationships or harmful life patterns if I think I know more than Jesus.

I handed my big sister, oldest daughter, know-it-all and holier-than-thou attitude to Jesus. Then I asked Him what do You give me in exchange? I was careful not to demand He give me something. I didn't barter with Him and say, "If I give You this will You give me something I want?" No, I just asked.

He gave me exactly what I needed and nothing more. He gave me Himself.

I wasn't exactly sure what He meant, so I asked. He let me know that I am a daughter of the King. He added, "There is safety in not having to be the boss." This response was crafted just for me.

For many years, I controlled everyone and everything around me out of fear of what would happen if I didn't and no one was in control. Now, Jesus was telling me, "It is OK, Father God and I have this. I'm walking with you, and He's protecting you. Your assignment is just to walk with Me."

There is such serenity in being a daughter of the King.

## ENDNOTES

1.  1 Samuel 16:23 NIV
2.  Philippians 2:9-11 NLT
3.  Philippians 4:13 NKJV

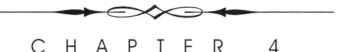

# SHAME

*"When God fulfills your longing, sweetness fills your soul."*

Proverbs 13:19 TPT

t was a late summer afternoon in the small community of five families where I grew up. Hide-and-go-seek was a game all of the kids could play. We ran easily between the front and back yards of the familiar houses finding new places to hide.

As one of the oldest, I was always first back to base and rarely had to be "it". This evening, though, I was it. The sun was going down to cool the heat of the day.

I was having a great time, not really worried about whether I could find everyone or not. I counted to 100 and then yelled, "Ready or not, here I come."

Out of the corner of my eye I saw Jimmy,[1] one of the younger boys, run around the corner. He saw me see him and knew he wouldn't be able to get away.

"Crisco, Crisco, fat in the can. You couldn't catch me no matter how fast you ran," he yelled laughing.

If he was trying to make me mad, it worked. If he was trying to get me to leave the game, that worked, too. If he was trying to make me ashamed, that worked as well. I stomped inside angry at the taunting of a three-year-old. I vowed never to play with the little kids again.

My brother and sister were still running, laughing and having a good time. While I marched into the house, they went on playing. That just made me feel they agreed with Jimmy. In essence, they probably didn't even hear him, and if they had, it wouldn't have registered as truth to them.

## I'M NOT FAT

I told myself I wasn't fat. In reality, I wasn't a chubby kid, but I sure felt fat. "Crisco, Crisco fat in the can" churned around and around in my head for decades after that incident.

It's interesting how some incidents trigger thoughts like, "I am fat. I am nothing". These thoughts then go through my conscious mind and are archived in my subconscious. They are categorized as emotions. Emotions can lie dormant for years, ready and waiting for any incident to retrieve it. These feelings are then expressed in actions.

I can be an intelligent, well-educated adult knowing exactly what I should eat, how I should move, the proper amount of restful activities and sleep I should get, and yet, something precludes me from taking care of myself. For some reason I am afraid to take time to understand what's going on deep inside.

Instead, I prefer to do harm to my body. It can be through any one of various means and methods. I chose overeating. I stuffed my emotions by trying to keep them quiet with food.

It's really difficult to understand how a mindless word rhyme coming out of a child's mouth could set off a ripple that years later would snowball into my weight gain of over 430 pounds.

It wasn't Jimmy's fault, though. Please do not misunderstand me. It was my perception, my negative self-image, which by age 11 was headed downhill fast.

## TRUTH

All lies are based on truth to some degree. I know I am not nothing. It's just that feelings speak louder than thoughts. My thoughts can be shifted by my emotions.

My feelings used Jimmy's words as a launching pad to build a wall of shame in my life. I was guilty of eating more than I should have, even as a kid. I'd sneak candy and cookies whenever I could.

My guilt turned into shame which said, "You are what you did. You are fat. You are shameful. You are a horrible donut monster."

My feelings take an element of truth and blow it completely out of proportion. If I nurse and feed it, it grows even more.

Shame followed me. I could never seem to shake it on my own. It was much later that I learned grace is the trump card which does away with shame. Jesus is the only one who can play the right card for me.

When I invited Jesus into my life, with Him came a grace I was totally ambivalent towards. As a child, I did not understand grace. I understood not burning in hell. Jesus was my fire insurance. That was pretty much the extent of my theology.

Once my salvation was settled, however, everything else seemed easy. I went to church, Sunday School, followed all the church rules as much as I could. I didn't worry about anything else except taking care of the situation at home. This consumed most of my time and all of my thoughts.

I did not understand that my older sister stance had relegated Jesus to the status of a kid playing outside.

As the big kid in our neighborhood, I wanted to shout, "Shut up," to little kids like Jimmy, who said things that made me want to cry. I wanted to make it a rule they couldn't talk.

## CAN I TALK TO YOU, JESUS?

Jesus relates in many ways to my siblings and early companions. I realize I silenced His voice in my life with my I-know-it-all attitude. I didn't want to listen to Him because He was like one of the little kids in the neighborhood who might say something mean without knowing it, or say something too close to the truth, which I couldn't handle. If I couldn't handle it, I would get angry, and anger was not an option. I saw anger as bad and not Christ-like.

Bottom line, I didn't want to hear what Jesus had to say. So, I shut off His voice. It took focusing on what my relationship was with Him before I saw this clearly. The next logical step was to understand if I had good communication with Jesus.

I asked Him, "Can I talk to you, Jesus? Is there a lie I am believing about how we communicate?"

In my mind I saw a picture of a strong Jesus enjoying life, walking with His disciples. Every now and again, He nodded to one of them as if He was carrying on a conversation. I was quite a ways behind Him, but I wanted to hear what He was saying. I began to run to catch up, but He got further and further away.

I called out to Him, "Jesus, wait. Jesus, it's me."

> I called out to Him, "Jesus, wait. Jesus, it's me."

He stopped, turned around and then, I saw it. He had a huge piece of duct tape across His mouth.

I stared at Him in disbelief. "Who did this to You?" I asked.

Immediately, I knew the answer. I hung my head. I looked up at Him.

"Jesus, it was me, wasn't it?"

All I wanted was the duct tape I had placed on my Savior's mouth to be removed. How to make that happen did not seem readily apparent. I felt like forgiving Jimmy was not necessary, but forgiving myself was. My reaction to not wanting to hear anything I deemed negative, whether it came from a little kid or Jesus, was a choice and I knew it. Just to be sure, I forgave Jimmy first.

"Jesus, I choose to forgive Jimmy for hurting my feelings even though I doubt he knew what he was doing. I renounce the lie You will hurt my feelings unknowingly, and not apologize or recognize You have done so. Jesus, what is Your truth?"

His answer was simple. "You know, I love you and I would never hurt you, ever."

I did know that, and I didn't really, even for one minute, think He would hurt me. That meant what I just prayed was for my own understanding. It was a first step in renewed communication between Jesus and me.

The duct tape had definitely come off His mouth. There was more to this process, and I knew what it was. I sighed, took a deep breath and exhaled. This would be hard.

"Jesus, I'm sorry for feeling I had a right to decide when I wanted to listen to Your voice and when I didn't. I was so very wrong for not listening when You would tell me things I didn't want to hear. I'm sorry for living for myself, and not for You. I'm sorry for playing like I was living for You when I really wasn't."

I continued. "Jesus, I renounce the lie You don't speak to me. I renounce the lie I can control Your voice. I renounce the lie You will tell me impossible things I can never do. I renounce the lie You will not help me accomplish the tasks which must be done for me to be whole, healthy and happy."

## The duct tape had definitely come off His mouth.

Complete forgiveness flooded over me. I knew there was nothing between Jesus and me at that moment. More than anything, I wanted to know what He would say to me next. "Jesus, what is Your truth for me?"

"Teresa, I love you with a love that is wider than the sea, deeper than the ocean, higher than the heavens. I speak to you all the time. I long more than anything for you to listen. I speak words of light and eternity all wrapped together. I speak words to lead you towards your destiny, purpose and calling.

56

"While on earth, I was fully man.[2] I know all your hurts, pains, temptations and trials. My voice and My words can help you navigate the treacheries which await you. Because I am also fully God,[3] I speak to Your heart. I speak words of life.[4]

"You have My words in My Word. Read them. Digest them daily.[5] Let them go deep into your soul. Let them wipe away the negative sea of words you have allowed to remain there. Let Me give you new words.[6] Let Me clean up your mind[7] and renew you, inside and out.[8]

"See, I am doing a new thing. Do you not see it? Do you not recognize it?[9] It is a new thing I am doing in your life. I have been revealing new things, hidden things, which will change your life.[10] As I reveal these things and you go through them we will become closer and closer, but only if you listen to My voice and follow Me.[11]

> Throughout the amazing events of those moments with Jesus, I understood more of what He was calling me to.

"The plans I share with you will move you forward to a destiny[12] and future you would never ask for or imagine.[13] What I have planned for you is far more than your mind can contain."

Through the amazing events of those moments with Jesus, I understood more of what He was calling me to. I was to spend more time not just reading, but really digesting, the words of Jesus as found in the Bible. I started with the book of John. I was amazed as words seemed to leap off the page.

I realized I had a know-it-all attitude about the Bible and Jesus. I have a college degree in Bible. I've been in church almost every Sunday of my life. I have a lot of head knowledge about what the Bible says about Jesus. However, what Jesus was calling me to was heart knowledge. It's different than applying what the Bible says, which is a "do" thing. I was moving past the self-effort scenario.

## DIGESTING HIS WORD

Jesus was calling me to meditate on His Word, not just know it, but to understand and let it grow in my heart.

Jesus told the Jewish leaders lots of things they didn't understand. His teaching in John 6 caused even some of His followers to turn away.

"I am the bread of life. Whoever comes to Me will never go hungry, and whoever believes in Me will never be thirsty ... I am the living bread which came down from heaven. If anyone eats of this bread, he will live forever; and the bread that I shall give is My flesh, which I shall give for the life of the world."[14]

The dividing point was this—those listening thought Jesus was telling them they would eat His flesh. They weren't understanding. He meant they should devour and digest His words. He means the same for me. God was telling me His words must be life to me. I was beginning to understand this truth on a new level.

What I needed was to be more enamored with His Word than I had been with food. As a recovering food addict, I identify with this. Before, I had always lived to eat high carbohydrate food—as much as I could eat, any time I could get it.

What if I lived to devour God's Word like I did food? What if I couldn't wait for the next meal Jesus hand-fed me? What if His Word was what sustained me each and every day? This breakthrough alone would be life-changing.

My interpretation of what Jesus said in John 6:35 is, "Come to me every day and you will never go hungry."[15] I wondered almost daily how I could weigh so much and still be hungry. I know now it is because I was eating the wrong things. Eating foods with high sugar and carbohydrate content only set up a reward cycle in my brain.

I would get a hit of sugar, whether from sugar or something else which converts to sugar in the bloodstream, and my brain immediately signaled it wanted more. Only the next time I had to have more than the time before.

If I put in the wrong food, all I got was fatter. If I put in the right food, I would become lean and fit. This is a simplified version, but it is an important truth.

> What if I lived to devour God's Word like I did food? What if I couldn't wait for the next meal Jesus hand-fed me? What if His Word was what sustained me each and every day?

Only the Word of God lasts, gives strength for the day and hope for tomorrow. I was always looking for the solution to my emotional turmoil in food. The truth is only God's Word has the real food I need to not only live, but to live in abundance. It has the words of real life.

There was still something in the way of me totally accepting God's Word as sustanance. It was the wall of shame. For years, all I could see was a barrier I built of the donuts, cakes and other sweets. I had constructed a giant barrier between Jesus and me and, therefore, between His Word and me.

It felt like He was jumping up and down, standing on His tippy toes, trying to peek over the mountain of junk foods, waving His arms and saying, "Hey, I'm over here. When you are ready, tell this wall to move, and it will. Then you can see Me completely."

Moving the wall, even if I could figure out how, was really scary because the space behind it had become my comfort zone. The wall, though, was not comfortable. The wall confined, enclosed and imprisoned me. It was a wall of my own making. The first step in it's removal was simply the desire to have it gone.

> The wall confined, enclosed and imprisoned me. It was a wall of my own making. The first step in it's removal was simply the desire to have it gone.

The proposition of removing this thing which had been a fixture in my life for as long as I could remember was overwhelming.

Jesus desires there to be nothing between me and Him.[16] I knew what the wall was made of. I also knew when I asked Him to help me remove the wall, I had to be willing to participate. I had to want the wall gone.

He was more than willing to remove the wall when I was. Was I ready? I was about to find out.

It's interesting how God works in my life. Years ago, He told me to give up sugar. He didn't say it just once, but many times. Why was this time different?

Maybe it was because God had to come in through the back door with His grace to rescue me. I've always had a solid connection with God, the Father. Because of watching my dad's dedication and faith walk, Father God was real to me in a special way.

## BACK DOOR OF GRACE

I had no problem of the concept of God as my Father. Jesus, however, was different. He should be my companion and communicator. He's the one who's lived here before. It stands to reason He would know how to get me out of the extreme weight quandary I had put myself in. Listening to His advice, though, made me want to quickly turn the channel.

By helping me understand the connection between alcohol and sugar, God came in through the only door I had open. My father was adamantly against alcohol because of alcoholism in his family. I had promised him I would never drink or be addicted.

When I began to understand I was like an alcoholic only with sugar, it was a strong connection to both my earthly father and Father God. I was ready to give up sugar because of my trust in God's leadership.

I was just beginning to accept Jesus' role in walking out my journey. He leads me and walks beside me. He's the Person of the Trinity who has been tempted in every way, just like I have, yet He didn't sin.[17]

Having Jesus guide me is so important. He resisted the temptation by the devil to turn stones to bread.[18] He was hungry. He had fasted for many days. No one would have faulted him for eating. Yet, He knew what the Father desired. What better guide than One who been tempted and who overcame the temptation?

## REMOVING THE WALL

Finally, I felt safe removing the wall of shame. So Father God and I removed the barrier of sugar, flour, cookies, breads, cakes, donuts, brownies, candies, chips and other junk food I had placed between Jesus and me.

As the wall came crashing down, each giant food item hit the ground and disintegrated into nothing. I sensed Jesus was standing beside me saying, "These things are nothing compared to the sweetness which will now be able to fill your soul."[19]

Where the wall once stood was a vast open field. There was no substance of shame behind the wall. There was nothing. The wall had been another lie shouting to me, "You don't deserve God's grace. You deserve His wrath. He is going to be so mad at you for what you've done. Run and hide behind this wall. Never come out again. Be ashamed." Now, the wall was gone.

This truth was very real as I stared into the field. There was no condemnation[20] here. Never again would I allow a wall of shame to define me. I will only allow Jesus to define me. I put my hand in His. We began walking, and He began talking. What He told me helped me understand more about who I am to Him. I would need this knowledge to continue my journey.

## ENDNOTES

1. Not his real name
2. Philippians 2:6-8 NIV
3. Philippians 2:9-11 NIV
4. John 6:63 NIV
5. John 6:35 NIV
6. Proverbs 25:11 NASB
7. Romans 12:2 NIV
8. Romans 12:1-2 MSG
9. Isaiah 43:19 NIV
10. Isaiah 48:6 NIV
11. John 10:27 NIV
12. Ephesians 2:10 TPT
13. Ephesians 3:20-21 NIV
14. John 6:35, 51 NIV
15. John 6:35 NLT
16. Romans 8:39 NIV
17. Hebrews 4:15 NIV
18. Matthew 4:3 NIV
19. Proverbs 13:19 TPT
20. Romans 8:1 NIV

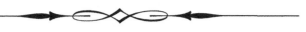

CHAPTER 5

# UNACCEPTED

*"It's God's own truth, nothing could be plainer: God plays no favorites! It makes no difference who you are or where you're from—if you want God and are ready to do as He says, the door is open."*

Acts 10:34 MSG

Talking to those assigned to our second grade lunch table, Bill[1] said, "I can't wait for Christmas morning," It was the last day before Christmas break. He added, "I think I'm getting a new bike."

"I love all the lights, the tree, the tinsel, the Santas," Sally[2] said with a dreamy look in her eyes. "My mom has the world's largest collection of Santa figurines."

"I love Santa Claus," I chimed in, thankful to have something I could talk about.

"You still believe in Santa Claus?" Bill's voice held a hint of disgust.

"Sure, he comes every year to my great-grandma's house."

"No, he doesn't."

"Yes, he does." My voice raised a bit at this point. I knew Santa came every year. There was no doubt in my mind.

"How do you know?" Sally said with a condescending smirk on her face. I didn't realize she was baiting me.

"Every Christmas Eve he comes to Mamaw's. We hear his bells when he comes around the house, and his 'Ho, Ho, Ho,' when he leaves the gifts by the front door. When we open it, there are the gifts." I was getting excited just thinking about it.

They were still laughing at me when the bell rang.

The entire table of second graders burst into laughter. Sally could barely contain herself as she explained, "There is no Santa Claus. It's just something adults make up to fool us."

"So how do the gifts get on the front porch?" I just couldn't let it go.

"Probably someone slips out the back door when you aren't looking, rings some bells, and leaves them on the porch," Bill said.

"What about at home? We go out to look at the Christmas lights, and when we get home, the presents are under the tree. Santa comes while we're doing that."

By this time, he was almost hysterical. "Your parents send you to the car and then put the presents under the tree. You're such a baby."

They were still laughing at me when the bell rang. They proceeded to play the game of gossip until the entire class knew I was a moron who still believed in Santa Claus.

I was angry. Why would my parents lie to me and leave me vulnerable to ridicule? I felt stupid arguing for the more childish belief side while all the others at my lunch table acted so much more mature.

When Dad got home, I confronted him about Santa Claus. To his credit, he explained the truth. He took the stance Santa Claus does exist in the spirit of giving at Christmas. He added the real meaning of Christmas about how Jesus came as a baby to live a sinless life, die and be resurrected.

Dad made me feel better, but still he and Mom lied to me, and then told me I couldn't tell my brother or other children about the lie.

Childhood is full of lies—Santa Claus, the Easter bunny, the tooth fairy and who knows what else? As a child, separating lies from truth is difficult. Separating intentional white lies meant in jest and fun is nearly impossible, even if the adult says they're, "Just kidding". A child never knows for sure.

This particular incident set up my fear of being unaccepted by those my age. I never wanted to go through such a situation again. I vowed to make sure I stayed on top of things, didn't voice my viewpoint and stayed quiet. I didn't want to risk not being accepted again.

## LIES

There came a time on my journey when I had gotten rid of enough lies to lose weight, but was concerned I might just put more weight back on again like I had time and time again. I wanted this time to be different. At any moment, an emotion I hadn't taken care of could rear its head, derail me and send me back to the way I was.

Then would I go back to what I call my "Plan B"? I knew God was Plan A, but would I ever go back to eating all the comfort foods I used to eat by the boat loads? How could I be sure I'd never do this again? I didn't want those thoughts, but they were there. I could not deny their existence.

I had pulled some deep emotional roots already. I hoped I was finished. Now, though, I knew I needed to embark on an even more intense journey than anything I had been on.

I was about to be thrown into a very different life. I had no idea I'd be speaking in public, doing television and radio interviews, coaching, shooting videos at least weekly and sometimes more, leading workshops and conducting study groups.

God knew my future, and He knew a lot of work had to be done before I was ready for this new level of freedom.

## HEALING EMOTIONS

I was interested in all types of inner healing because I knew my emotions were basically a hodgepodge of many misconceptions. I did not realize how the things I experienced as a child affected even my beliefs about God.

By this time, I had lost the physical weight. I had learned a lot about myself, and challenged many of the lies I believed. I followed many wonderful Bible teachers, especially Joyce Meyer, Beth Moore and Henry Blackaby. I'd been to counselors, conferences and seminars. I'd read many self-help books, and taken every psychological, strengths, spiritual gifts, personality and motivations test around.

I had already done a lot of work. However, I knew there was more work to be done. I had a quest for wholeness. As a triune being, I am a body, a soul and a spirit. I wanted every part of me to work together. I wanted to be whole, healthy and happy.

## THE BASIS FOR FREEDOM

Real freedom started for me when I began to understand the connections between perceptions I had from childhood and emotional triggers which influenced how I felt about God.

Why does how I feel about God matter? Isn't God, God? How I feel about Him doesn't change Him. It doesn't change who God is, but it does change how I believe in, adhere to, trust in, rely on and have faith[3] in Him. The more I know God as God instead of a conglomerate I have created, the freer I will become.

I accepted Jesus as my Savior when I was seven. My father was a preacher. There wasn't too much I didn't know about the Bible. It was in my head, but it needed to move to my heart, and then, to my feet to be walked every day. This is what it means to be made new.[4]

Each day I am being made new. It is ongoing. I should not stay the same at the same level of understanding and knowledge I had when I came to Christ as a child. I am changed into His image again and again or "from glory to even more glory."[5]

How does that happen? It happens by the Spirit of the Lord when I behold the glory of the Lord. This means I must continually seek Him in order to "progressively be transformed".[6] Somewhere along the line, I had stopped seeking and just began to amass knowledge. I thought I knew it all and had heard it all. It's a dangerous place to stop, right on the edge of moving from crawling to soaring.

As a child, things occurred which I had no ability to process at the time. I processed the best I could. My perceptions went into the filter of my brain at five, eight, 11 or 15 and came out as a lie. They were lies I didn't recognize. However, they were lies I believed.

How do I un-believe what I have believed? It is a process of uncovering truth. It comes by the fact that "the Lord is the Spirit, and where the Spirit of the Lord is, there is liberty emancipation from bondage, true freedom."[7]

# THE PROCESS

As a super morbidly obese woman for much of my life, I had a difficult time believing God accepted me. The lack of acceptance, though, felt like it had always been with me. It became worse as I got larger. Up until that time most of my life was spent trying to get God's acceptance.

Understanding the depths of this, amazingly, went back to sitting at the lunch table with a bunch of too-smart second graders, who made me feel like an outcast because I believed in Santa Claus. In reality, though, it wasn't their actions which made me feel unaccepted by God, it was learning my father had not told me the truth.

The little girl me believed I wasn't accepted as smart enough to know the truth. I was upset with Dad, which I couldn't express and simply stuffed the pain and frustration down inside.

As the oldest child, I thought my parents would always tell me the truth. When I learned I'd been duped, it was difficult to take. As a child I could cognitively accept Dad's explanation, but still he lied to me.

Accepting the rational side of the situation is one thing, but the emotional side of me blamed Dad for the other kids laughing at me. I could still hear their laughter echoing in my head. Even though Dad did nothing wrong emotionally I was wounded, and I saw it as his fault. More than all of this, it related to me not feeling accepted by Father God.

The process is simple. I forgave Dad by just stating this to Father God. It was an acceptance of the emotionally wounded seven-year-old who still governed a part of my feelings.

I said, "I forgive Dad for not telling me the truth about Santa Claus. I forgive him for making the lie so believable I challenged the other second graders, and made myself look ridiculous. I forgive Dad for not accepting I was old enough to understand the truth."

Because how I feel about my earthly father relates to how I feel about God, I renounced the lie Father God will treat me the same way. "I renounce the lie You, Father God, don't accept me as a person who can understand the truth. I

> I could still hear their laughter echoing in my head.

renounce the lie You will intentionally upset me. I renounce the lie You will make me look ridiculous by allowing me to believe something childish about You. I renounce the lie You don't accept me as a person of worth and destiny. Now, Father God, what is Your truth?"

Truth is not easily discerned in every instance in everyday life. However, I've found when I ask God a direct question it's like He's sitting on the edge of His throne eager to communicate with me.

Going through this process has helped me understand so much more of how prayer works. It's communication with God. What do we have to talk to Him about? We talk to Him about Himself. He is always ready to share truth with me. Always.

## GOD'S TRUTH

When God answers me, whether through a thought, a picture or a feeling, I write it down as soon as I can, preferably at the same time. I want to remember what He said to me, what I sensed or saw. Then I test the revelation through Scripture.

I asked God, "What is Your truth?" I heard Him speaking in my mind.,"I love you. More than that, I like you, Teresa Shields Parker. I created you with a specific purpose.[8] I recreated you to fulfill this destiny.[9] Each experience you have gone through in your life is a part of My plan for you.[10] It's a piece in the puzzle. I'm giving you all the pieces.

"This issue of rebelling against Me, gaining an enormous amount of weight, nearly killing My creation which is you, is all forgiven. It's gone. I remember it no more.[11] You, however, are having a hard time forgetting.

"It is foundational in your journey and makes you unique, but it does not define you. I define you. Your connection to Me defines you. My love defines you. My presence in your life leading you forward defines you.

"Never forget this, Teresa Shields Parker, I created you.[12] You are mine."[13]

The fact He called me by name, not once but twice, just reinforces His specific love for me.

I am also aware of the name He used for me. This is my professional name, my author, coach and speaker name. It is my maiden name and married name together. It says to me, this is how He sees me now, just like I am. This in and of itself, if He said nothing else to me, speaks of monumental acceptance and destiny.

The song, "Just As I Am" was one we sang every Sunday at church. I memorized the words, but I really hadn't experienced the truth of them. I wondered as a child, did God really accept me with all my imperfections?

Now, the truth of His acceptance was deep in my heart. God accepts me no matter who I am or what I have done. He accepted, loved and forgave me. I know He will do the same for anyone else. We have all failed,[14] but His door is still open to us.

> God accepts me no matter who I am or what I have done.

"It's God's own truth, nothing could be plainer: God plays no favorites! It makes no difference who you are or where you're from—if you want God, and are ready to do as He says, the door is open."[15]

No one is exempt from God's love,[16] but everywhere I turn I find people who feel they are the exception to this promise from God. They feel their ability to overindulge in sweets and gain an extreme amount of weight is unforgivable. Nothing could be further from the truth.

There is a place of sweet freedom. There is a place of forgiveness. For a long time, I did not believe even if I lost weight, God could forgive me for what I had done to my body. Before I can forgive anyone else, I must believe I am forgiven. It's not an easy journey, but it's one which must be taken for freedom to grow.

## EXCHANGE PROCESS

I dragged a huge bag loaded with concrete blocks of shame, anger and frustration with me everywhere I went. These were by-products of being ridiculed and feeling unaccepted. As an adult, I realized it was my choice to hold on to these feelings. In other words, I did this to myself.

I stayed in shame even after losing most of my weight. Going through pictures of me when I was close to my highest weight, I found the before picture I use today. The day it was taken, I was ashamed. There was no place for me to hide. No one to hide behind. No wall to peek around.

It was me carrying all 430 pounds marked with anger, depression, shame, guilt, frustration, hopelessness, control, defeat, anger, hunger, self-effort, lack of acceptance and so much more. Each pound had an emotional tag.

I began identifying the feelings. As I handed each one to God, I asked His forgiveness for carrying the particular feeling and the weight it represented. As I gave each to God, He gave me gifts like love, joy, peace, patience, kindness, goodness, faithfulness, gentleness and self-control.[17]

I identified more—rebellion, self-sufficiency, fear, loneliness, hunger, mistrust. As I handed each to God, He gave me mercy, grace, contentment, wisdom, compassion, encouragement and courage.

It was an exhilarating experience. Losing physical weight is wonderful. Many things change just because of being thinner, such as having more energy and stamina. However, sweet freedom for me came at handing each piece of emotional baggage to Him and receiving a gift in exchange.

> Sweet freedom for me came at handing each piece of emotional baggage to Him and receiving a gift in exchange.

It's not a singular event, though. As other embedded lies, strongholds and damaged emotions become known to me, I again go through this simple process of handing them to God and asking Him, "What do You give me in exchange?" I do so love His gifts.

His gifts are meant to lead me to freedom and they did. However, there was still more sweet freedom ahead. I was about to learn deeper truths about why the foods I crave can never fill the vast emptiness inside.

## ENDNOTES

1. Not his real name
2. Not her real name
3. John 6:29 AMP
4. 2 Corinthians 5:17 NLT
5. 2 Corinthians 3:18 AMP
6. ibid.
7. 2 Corinthians 3:17 AMP
8. Psalm 139:16 NLT
9. Ephesians 2:10 TPT
10. Romans 8:28 NIV
11. Isaiah 43:25 NIV
12. Psalm 139:13-16 NLT
13. Isaiah 43:1 NIV
14. Romans 3:23 NIV
15. Acts 10:34 MSG
16. John 3:16 NIV
17. Galatians 5:22-23 NLT

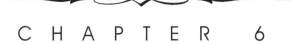

CHAPTER 6

# HUNGER

*"For I'm trained in the secret of overcoming
all things, whether in fullness or in hunger. And
I find the strength of Christ's explosive power
infuses me to conquer every difficulty."*

Philippians 4:11-13 TPT

W e were standing in the kitchen of my grandparents two-story farmhouse. It was a room which oozed love from every corner, especially if my favorite person in all the world was there as well.

"Can we make cookies now?" I asked.

Grandma smiled and gave me a hug. "Surely, you know making cookies with you is my favorite-ist thing in the whole world to do." She wore a dress with pink and black geometric designs on it. She sewed her everyday dresses just alike. They had round necklines, short sleeves, waists and full skirts.

"Your dress is pretty," I said. I reached up to hug her around the middle. She had soft, mushy parts just right for hugging. In my mind, her larger than life size was because of the love which poured out of her and into me.

"OK, let's get the ingredients together for our secret oatmeal cookie recipe. I'll get the butter. You get the sugar, baking soda, baking powder, salt, vanilla and our secret ingredient." She winked as she pulled the kitchen step stool up to the counter for me.

From as far back as I can remember, making cookies with Grandma was a treat. Of course, I loved eating them warm from the oven, but more than that, I loved working with Grandma and learning from her.

## THE RECIPE

At seven, I pretty much knew the recipe by heart. I'm sure some of allowing me to get the ingredients together had to do with teaching me the recipe.

"Wash your hands first. Then get the sugars ready," she said.

I did as she instructed, measuring the white sugar and poured it into the bowl, then the brown sugar.

"What's next?" she asked.

"One cup of butter," I said.

"Measure it carefully."

I scooped the butter out into the measuring cup and into the bowl with the sugars. Using a huge spoon, I began to stir the ingredients together. It was hard. I had to stop several times because my arm got tired.

"Here, I'll give it a go while you rest." She took an oversize tablespoon and began whipping the butter and sugar together until I couldn't tell they had once been separate ingredients. It was amazing.

"Can I crack the eggs, Grandma?"

"No, you don't know how yet."

"Sure I do. I watch you all the time."

Just then the phone rang with two short rings and a long one. Grandma was on a party line, but this was her ring.

"Here, stir the dough while I get the phone. It's probably the club president. I need to talk to her."

It was easier to stir now. I loved the creamy texture. The more I stirred the more my desire to taste the cookies rose. Grandma was talking low and quiet. Her head was turned towards the wall.

I reached for an egg from the pottery bowl on the counter. Grandma would be so proud of me when she saw I had made the entire batch of cookies while she was talking important business. I was a big girl. I knew how.

## CRACKING THE EGG

I gave the egg a good crack on the side of the cabinet like I'd seen Grandma do hundreds of times, but instead of staying in one half of the shell like Grandma's always did, it ran down the side of the cabinet and landed in a plop on the floor.

"Teresa, why on earth did you do that?" Grandma quickly apologized to the person on the phone and hung up. "What did I tell you?"

"I ... I wanted to surprise you. I wanted to finish the cookies."

"Well, it certainly is a surprise to have egg all over the kitchen floor."

She stood looking back and forth from the floor to me. I could tell she was upet. When Mom got mad, I always got a spanking and it really hurt. I deserved one. I knew that. Would Grandma spank me? I didn't know if I could stand it if she did. I could hardly stand her being angry with me.

"Come with me." She took me by the hand and marched me through the kitchen, down the long dining room, through the living room, where the door upstairs stood in one corner, down the hall to the bathroom. "Stay in there until I come back for you."

## SCARED TO BE ALONE

The minute she shut the door, I started scream-crying. It wasn't because I was sad. I was scared to be alone. I never went in that part of the house by myself.

Then, I remembered. There was a second door out of the bathroom into the dining room. It was always locked with a hook at the top of the door, but on the bathroom side. All I had to do was climb up on the toilet, unlatch the door and I was back in the kitchen in no time.

Grandma was cleaning the egg mess off the cabinet when I came running in. "Oh no, you don't. You and I both need some time apart." She marched me back down to the bathroom. This time she locked both doors from the outside.

I spent my time in the bathroom, all five minutes of it, wailing. It seemed like eons before she came. I was sure she hated my guts and would never speak to me again. I'd spoiled everything because I disobeyed.

When she let me out, she sat down in the big chair in the living room and pulled me up on her lap. Her voice was kind and sweet.

"Teresa, I'm sorry for getting mad at you, and I'm sorry for leaving you in the bathroom. I needed some time to get over being upset, and it was the only place I could think of to put you until I could calm down."

"Grandma, I'm sorry for cracking the egg. I thought I knew how, and I just wanted to finish the cookies 'cause I wanted to eat some."

"Cracking an egg is the hardest part about baking cookies," she said. "There's a knack to it. It's hard to explain, but I can teach you."

I reached up, hugged her and gave her a kiss on the cheek. "I love you, Grandma."

"Honey, if you loved me half as much as I love you, it'd be enough."

She was the one person in the world I loved with everything in me. So, if that was half of the way she loved me, I was monstrously loved.

## THE WAY WE ATE

Any time we went to my grandmother's house for a family dinner there was a spread which looked like it was meant to feed a crew of 20 hard-working farm hands. This was true even if it was just our family of five and my grandparents.

The fact they lived on a farm and were both raised in generational farm families dictated the predominance of starchy foods and desserts on my grandmother's table. She couldn't cook any other way. Meals were her job. Papaw worked in the field, tended the animals, took care of the farm machinery and kept the books.

Grandma planted and tended the garden. She gathered the green beans, potatoes, peas, corn, tomatoes, cucumbers and other vegetables. Then, she cooked, canned or froze them. She fed the chickens and gathered the eggs. Papaw would milk the cow and bring the fresh milk up each morning.

She would prepare all the meals, plus churn butter and make cottage cheese and bake bread, cakes, cookies and hoecakes. When it was time for fried chicken, she'd choose several, kill them, pluck them, cut them up into pieces and fry them.

She and Papaw ran the farm like a well-oiled machine. Everything they did revolved around making sure there was more than enough for everyone to eat.

## INHERITANCE OF FOOD

It's no wonder, then, when Grandma died in 1993 and Mom, six months before her, the main thing I inherited was boxes and boxes of recipes.

The recipes went further back than Grandma because as the oldest daughter, she had inherited her mother's recipes. I am the oldest daughter of the oldest daughter of the oldest daughter. Holding the recipe boxes in my hands felt as if I was holding the lifeblood of our family. All our cultural traditions seemed to center around food.

Looking through the recipes, I began to understand why my family ate the way they did. I always thought we had a unique gene which made us hungry all the time. My grandparents and ancestors were farmers, laboring long hours. They needed an overabundance of high calorie energy to do the work they did.

Big family dinners were held for birthdays, holidays and any special, or not so special, occasion. There were family reunions on every side. Each great aunt could have won the state fair baking contest. I lived for family get-togethers.

**Fat and happy seemed to be our family motto.**

Fat and happy seemed to be our family motto. I certainly didn't want to be the one to curtail the full, satisfied and content feeling. I loved eating all of the foods I grew up with. I didn't have a thought about not eating them.

Today, I live in a different era where I, like many others, sit and stare at a computer screen all day. I don't need the calories my ancestors needed just to survive.

There came a point on my weight loss journey when I felt I had a barrier in the way of me losing any more weight. I wasn't anywhere near my goal, but I was stuck.

It felt scary to even touch a pound below where I was. It was like dipping my foot in water which might be electrically charged. I'd touch it and shrink back.

There was a wall which needed to be gone, but I had no idea what it was. I also knew if I couldn't figure it out, I would be stuck there forever.

I shared this in a group meeting. Others gave me input, but nothing was registering. Then my mentor asked me a question which seemed totally unrelated to what I had just shared. "Where did you learn your relationship with food?"

The question invaded my mind. Not for a second did I wonder if I had a relationship with food. I knew I did, and I knew I learned it from Grandma.

## Where did you learn your relationship with food?

My mother, having taken home economics in high school, tried to plan balanced meals. She did not cook tons of food for seconds. We had a small refrigerator. She wanted nothing leftover.

If there were five at the table, there would be five pieces of meat or servings of the main dish. There would be vegetables and something starchy, like potatoes or noodles. Dessert would be a can of peaches or fruit cocktail divided among those at the table.

As a kid, I preferred Grandma's more lavish style of cooking. She'd always try to cook each person's favorite dish if she could. I wasn't a big fish-eater. So, when it came time for the catfish fry, she'd be sure to have fried potatoes and hoecake, a fried white cornbread, because those were my favorites. Of course, there would always be many desserts to choose from.

I equated the kind of foods Grandma prepared with comfort and love. When I was away from her and felt overwhelmed, sad, angry, lonely, fearful, worried, stressed or just plain old frustrated, I would make something Grandma would have made. It was my comfort food. It would comfort for a while until the sugar-high wore off, and I needed more.

This way of coping wasn't comforting at all. It was very discomforting. In reality it was killing me.

Still, to not eat or cook those foods felt like I would be abandoning my culture and dishonoring Grandma. It took me awhile to process what was happening in my head and heart.

To believe Grandma's foods, which were my favorites, had been harming me, saddened me. I knew she didn't aim to hurt me. She fed me out of love. However, the little girl in me was emotionally attached to those comfort foods, which equaled extreme love. While the adult me knew I couldn't eat all of those foods in the quantities I was consuming them and be healthy, the emotional part of me was still stuck back baking cookies with Grandma.

## THE FOOD WALL

In essence, Grandma's cooking was the wall. Grandma wasn't the barrier, but her cooking was. I had equated the two. They had become enmeshed in my heart. Could I separate them? Could I still hold a place in my heart for Grandma if I turned my back on the things she cooked?

My great-grandmother's oatmeal cake, which Grandma baked often, was one of my favorites. It was part of my heritage. So was the tub of oatmeal cookies, which was always in the lowest cupboard so grandchildren could help themselves. I couldn't imagine never again having hot rolls, chocolate pie, brownies or myriads of other special dishes.

The emotional wall of cultural foods was vivid in my mind. They emanated from Grandma's kitchen and the kitchens of my wonderful female ancestors, who each had specialties we looked forward to consuming at each family get together.

After sharing what I had discovered, my mentor asked, "What would your grandmother say to you if she knew certain foods were causing you to ruin your health?"

## Clearly, though, it was true. Mom had the better way.

I knew she would tell me to give them up. Many times she would say to me, "Honey, you would feel so much better if you would lose some weight." However, about five minutes later, she would say, "I baked a batch of oatmeal cookies. They're in the cabinet. Eat as many as you want." Of course, I would. The second message drowned out the first.

I clearly saw the disconnect between these two statements. I also realized she never saw it. She was a large woman, but never as large as me. She ate what she needed, but she also worked hard in the garden, tending the chickens, carrying laundry to and from the basement, hanging it to dry, ironing and cleaning house. She rarely sat, but when she did she usually had a bucket of peas to shell or green beans to break. It never dawned on her certain foods could be addictive.

During the group meeting, I let those foods go and I embraced more of what my mother had been trying to teach me. Part of me didn't want to agree she had been trying to teach me a better way than Grandma.

Grandma was my person. Mom was just someone who acted crazy for most of my growing up years. Clearly, though, it was true. Mom had the better way.

## FORGIVE MYSELF

I was thankful for this insight, but during my quiet time I knew the first thing I had to do was forgive myself for not learning the lessons of limited, practical, balanced meals my mother had been trying to teach me.

As a kid, I thought she was being mean by limiting what we ate and telling us we had to eat the vegetables, or horror of horrors, the liver and onions, before we got dessert, which was part of a can of peaches. I forgave myself and thanked my mother, who was in the great beyond by this time, for trying to teach me some life-saving truths.

I confessed to the Holy Spirit I was sorry for not listening to what He had been trying to teach me many years ago when He revealed giving up sugar and breads and eating meats, fruits and vegetables was the way to walk out of the food prison I had put myself in.

## FORGIVE GRANDMA

I also forgave Grandma. It felt silly to forgive her. However, I knew it was necessary to tell the little girl who was still inside me that the adult me understood her emotional attachment to those foods. The adult me understood these comfort foods had formed a cultural barrier to weight loss. The little girl me needed to know the adult me understood the emotions, which seemed to hold me back every time I tried to go forward.

I said out loud, "Holy Spirit, I forgive Grandma for feeding me wonderful foods which would become addictive to me. I forgive her for making me feel food equals love and comfort. I understand she would be sad to know what these types of food did to me. I know she did not mean to hurt me."

Then, I renounced the lie, the Holy Spirit would comfort me in a way which would be harmful to me. I asked, "Holy Spirit, what is Your truth?"

I really didn't hear or sense words. I simply felt love and peace invade my being, like being swaddled in a warm, secure blanket. I understood, for the first time, this is what real comfort feels like. It's not an overfull feeling, which leads to damaging my body. It is a peace like only the Holy Spirit brings.

Jesus said this to His disciples. "But the Helper, Comforter, Advocate, Intercessor, Counselor, Strengthener, Standby, the Holy Spirit, whom the Father will send in My name, in My place, to represent Me and act on My behalf, He will teach you all things. And He will help you remember everything that I have told you.

I understood for the first time, this is what real comfort feels like.

"Peace I leave with you; My perfect peace I give to you; not as the world gives do I give to you. Do not let your heart be troubled, nor let it be afraid. Let My perfect peace calm you in every circumstance and give you courage and strength for every challenge."[1]

Knowing the Holy Spirit brings with Him a myriad of resources encouraged me. Knowing He is Comforter and Guide throughout my life, and specifically on this health journey, is a truth I cling to with everything in me.

When I am fully aware of the abiding presence of the Holy Spirit, I will be content and at peace no matter what the circumstance. It's when I'm not content that striving and trying in my own strength tries to take over. When this happens, I'm sure to fail.

"I have learned to be satisfied with whatever I have. I know what it means to lack and I know what it means to experience overwhelming abundance. For I'm trained in the secret of overcoming all things, whether in fullness or in hunger. And I find the strength of Christ's explosive power infuses me to conquer every difficulty."[2]

> If I am satisfied, it means I am at peace. I am fully engaged with what the Holy Spirit is doing in my life.

If I am satisfied, it means I am at peace. I'm fully engaged with what the Holy Spirit is doing in my life. I am constantly aware of where my power comes from. It's not from foods I crave. It's from Christ and Him alone.

I can live without comfort foods. However, I can't live without the Comforter's abiding presence, perfect peace and explosive power. What can I do with His explosive power? God was teaching me, the sky is not even the limit.

ENDNOTES

1.  John 14:26-27 AMP
2.  Philippians 4:11-13 TPT

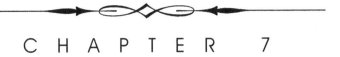

# CHAPTER 7

# MOVE

*"Strip down, start running—and never quit! No extra spiritual fat, no parasitic sins. Keep your eyes on Jesus, who both began and finished this race we're in. Study how He did it. Because He never lost sight of where He was headed—that exhilarating finish in and with God."*

Hebrews 12:1-2 MSG

I walked into the grade school gym, keeping my place in line. There suspended from the ceiling was the ominous rope. I literally felt myself getting sick. Actually, getting sick would be preferable to trying to climb the rope.

It was useless and pointless for me to even try. I had never gotten even a foot off the ground. The girls would snicker. The boys would laugh out loud. I'd only seen boys climb to the top of the ceiling where we were supposed to be able to reach. Most of the athletic girls could get to the top of the gym teacher's head before dropping off.

I hated the yearly fitness exam, and I especially hated the rope. It represented my complete failure in the way of Physical Education. Climbing the rope was a big portion of the grade. By sixth grade, the teacher would ask, "Do you want to try?"

"Do I have to?"

"Not if you can't climb over a foot. The grade is the same either way."

"Thanks," I'd say as I walked away.

I wasn't a fat kid, but I was uncoordinated, and hated physical exercise of any kind. Since I didn't exercise, run or play much at home, my muscles had no strength.

I could walk, though. Walking the mile was something I couldn't avoid. We had to walk around the gym for the duration of the class or until we completed a mile. This seemed to last forever.

There was no opting out of the mile walk. Every score counted into our class average. Perhaps I was just lazy, but it seemed pointless to walk around and around the gym a zillion times to get a little mark of completion. I did it, but I was not happy about it.

These two feats, though, weren't the only portions of the test. There were sit-ups and pushups. I could do the sit-ups, but pushups were impossible.

> I wasn't a fat kid, but I was uncoordinated and hated physical exercise of any kind.

The monkey bars, which looked like a ladder strung between two ladders, wasn't any fun. We were required to climb the ladder and then, swing hand over hand to the next ladder. I could never climb the ladder. So, that was out for me.

In high school, P.E. was a requirement, but only every other day. Still, it was my least favorite class, and the one in which

I got the lowest grade. If I showed up, I got at least a C, but I wanted all A's.

To get a better grade, I had to excel to some degree. The only sport I enjoyed and excelled at even remotely was swimming. Luckily we had a pool. Only half of the semester would be devoted to swimming. Since there were two semesters a year, I still could never hope to get anywhere near an A in P.E.

Basically the only class I hated was P.E. The only good to come out of it was I discovered I loved the water. Other than that, exercise was spelled t-o-r-t-u-r-e.

## DIET AND EXERCISE

Years later, I went on one of my many diet kicks, and exercise was a requirement. The program had a list of suggested exercises. One of them was water aerobics. Since I had always liked swimming, I thought it might be a good fit.

Employees where I worked got a discount on a water aerobics class at a local gym. I decided to brave finding a swimsuit in my size and joining. At 350 pounds I knew I would stand out, but I was committed to following the program.

I expected to feel embarrassed and humiliated the first day of class. To my surprise there were several women my size and larger in the class. I was even able to keep up with the instructor.

I enjoyed the six-week session. The next session, though, was over my budget, and I had to stop. I had lost some weight combining diet and exercise, but once again I threw in the towel. It did take a lot of time, an hour after work right at the time I should be cooking supper for my family. I told myself I would try the old exercise bike turned clothes rack, but I never did.

Fast forward about 10 more years and we had decided to take in foster children. Two of the girls we had were large. Their counselor wanted them to start exercising.

Our community had a nice recreation center complete with a large pool, track, exercise equipment, exercise bikes and basketball court. My own children were teenagers and looked forward to using the center, so we got a reasonably-priced family membership.

I also noticed free water aerobics classes were offered with the membership. By this time, I was nearing my highest weight. It was more difficult to complete the class because I was busy doing freelance writing and publishing. I made it to the class several times a month, but I was far from a regular attender.

## The rhythm of the water was soothing.

Through the years, I'd have on-again, off-again spurts of attending water aerobics. If I had to exercise, anything in the water was my choice. Still I hadn't convinced myself the time, energy and effort was worth it.

Several times when I arrived late to class, I noticed individuals walking or running around the water walking track, which some call the lazy river. Since I was already in my suit, I thought why not try it? As it turned out, I loved walking around the track. The rhythm of the water was soothing.

It also freed up additional times I could choose to be in the pool. I didn't have to get to the pool at the specific time a class started. I could make my own class. I still hadn't gotten to the place where I really saw a lot benefit from exercise, but I was doing a little.

It would take a true moment of change to get me to the place where I not only saw the benefit to exercise, but began to embrace it as a part of my life. Interestingly enough it coincided with understanding what foods were holding me back on my journey.

## STOP-START

About this time, my mentor introduced me to the concept of stop-start. This simple way of changing a negative habit into a positive became my go-to method of moving forward.

The basic premise is this. In my brain I have neural pathways, which are like shortcuts I establish. For instance, I have a neural pathway, which says brush my teeth in the morning and evening. My brain doesn't have to think about it. It just automatically leads me to do it.

In the same way, I have neural pathways established regarding bad habits. I can't just do away with those. If I want to change a bad habit, I have to overwrite the neural pathway with a good habit.

I stop the bad habit, and start the good one in its place. I put firm boundaries around the bad, and focus on the good. After my moment of change, at the next group meeting, my mentor asked me, "What are you going to focus on this week?"

I knew he was asking what would I stop and what would I start. This would be my first stop-start. Remembering that sugar is one molecule away from alcohol, I wanted to say,

"I'm going to stop eating sugar." However, I also wanted to be successful. I felt stopping all sugar would be too big of a bite to take at first.

So, I said, "I'm going to stop eating candy." Candy is very identifiable. I know what it is. There is no doubt if something is candy or not. Candy is what I would stop.

"What will you start?" he asked.

## STARTING EXERCISE

Out of my mouth came, "I'm going to start exercise." It sort-of surprised me. Even with just a haphazard approach to water exercise I had gotten benefit from it. Also it was an exercise I could do and not hurt. I had no idea if this would work with the neural pathway thing, but my mentor seemed to have no problem with it.

What he did have a problem with was my non-specific, generalized statement. "What type of exercise will you do?"

"I'm going to walk in the water."

"Where, when and how often will you do this?"

He was getting pretty picky with his specifics. I had to think. "I'll do it at the recreation center where the pool is. I'll do it three times a week during the morning."

"For how long?"

"Oh, 30 minutes."

"When?"

"Whenever I can."

He paused and looked at me. "How do you know when you have to get to an appointment, like a doctor's appointment or coming to this group meeting?"

I wasn't sure what he meant, but I said, "I put it in my iCalendar so I have it on my phone and computer."

"Then, make an appointment with yourself and keep it just like you'd keep any other appointment."

So, I did. I began the next day. Although I said three days a week, I found I enjoyed it so much I began going five days a week.

When I chose to stop candy and start exercise, I wasn't sure if the two would work together, but they did. I realized I had been eating candy by the bagsful because of several reasons. I was bored. I was fatigued. I needed energy, and I thought candy gave it to me. It was a habit.

Water exercise met all of those needs. I was no longer bored. I had a specific thing to do outside of my home. Working from home, even when I was doing something I loved, got boring. Exercise broke up the day and gave me something to look forward to. Exercise gave me the kind of energy I needed. After exercising I felt invigorated and alive. Plus, it didn't have the energy spike and the severe drop eating sugar does. Candy was pretty much straight sugar. Now, I was no

> I was bored. I was fatigued. I needed energy, and I thought candy gave it to me. It was a habit. Water exercise met all those needs.

longer fatigued during the day. I was tired at night, and slept better than I had in a long time.

Pretty soon, I was running in the water for an hour a day, many times six days a week. Plus, I found another wonderful benefit of exercise besides losing weight. I had time to meditate and listen to God. With no electronic devices to capture me, He had my full attention.

Some of my best prayer and conversation times with God are in the water. It is another reason I look forward to my exercise time and am sad if I have a day when I'm gone or can't work in the time.

Fortunately, the pool is open from early until late so I can usually find a time to exercise. Now exercise is a highlight of my day.

## WHOLE EXERCISE

During one of my times in the water, God began talking to me about the reason exercise is necessary for Christians. He explained He wants fit soldiers for His Kingdom.

It won't do any good to lose weight if I am still not strong and not in shape. I can't run the race He requires of me. It's a really big deal to God for us to pay attention to our bodies. It's His dwelling place on earth.

"Don't you realize that your body is the temple of the Holy Spirit, who lives in you and was given to you by God? You do not belong to yourself, for God bought you with a high price. So you must honor God with your body."[1]

He lives in me. I'm His home. I wouldn't let my home get run-down, holes in the roof, foundation shaky and walls crumbling. Yet, I found myself in this very condition. I was out of shape, physically, emotionally and spiritually. I needed exercise for every part of my body.

The writer of Hebrews says it this way. "Strip down, start running—and never quit! No extra spiritual fat, no parasitic sins. Keep your eyes on Jesus, who both began and finished this race we're in. Study how He did it. Because He never lost sight of where He was headed—that exhilarating finish in and with God—He could put up with anything along the way: Cross, shame, whatever.

"And now He's there, in the place of honor, right alongside God. When you find yourselves flagging in your faith, go over that story again, item by item, that long litany of hostility He plowed through. That will shoot adrenaline into your souls!"[2]

I have to understand I am in a race, not only for my life, but for the lives of others around me who desperately need my Savior. The real purpose of my life isn't my comfort and happiness. The real purpose of this life is to follow the will of God. Many times this will mean I have to give up the things I think I love for the One worth living for.

## WE'RE IN A RACE

"Do you not know that in a race all the runners run, but only one gets the prize? Run in such a way as to get the prize. Everyone who competes in the games goes into strict training. They do it to get a crown that will not last, but we do it to get a crown that will last forever. Therefore, I do not run like someone running aimlessly; I do not fight like a boxer beating the air. No, I strike a blow to my body and make it my slave so that after I have preached to others, I myself will not be disqualified for the prize."[3]

As I read these verses, I realized if I were running in a race I would come in last place. In the beginning, when I started exercising, I'd be walking slowly around the track. Everyone, even the older ladies would pass me. I longed to be able to walk faster. Running, though, was my dream.

> Exercise has become a springboard not only to weight loss, but to a lifetime of keeping the weight where it needs to be.

Now I run around the water track. I still can't do it on land, but maybe one day I will. It, too, is a dream of mine. Just suffice it to say, disobedience to God and carrying 260 extra pounds of weight on my body for years has taken its toll. I may never be the fastest person or be able to walk the longest distance. However, I'm farther along today, than I was yesterday, but not as far along as I will be tomorrow.

Moving used to be a barrier for me on my weight loss journey. All it took for me was understanding I can begin somewhere. I can move. Now, exercise has become a springboard not only to weight loss, but to a lifetime of keeping the weight where it needs to be. It is possible because I love the feeling of being healthier, and just being able to move easier.

I'm committed to this race called life because God is the giver of life. He gave me a choice. "Today I have given you the choice between life and death, between blessings and curses. Now I call on heaven and earth to witness the choice you make. Oh, that you would choose life, so that you and your descendants might live! You can make this choice by loving the Lord your God, obeying Him, and committing yourself firmly to Him."[4]

I'm choosing life. It's really the only choice.

Sometimes in choosing life, fear of not being protected hits, seemingly out of the blue. Where does it come from and how can I move past it? Only with the help of the Father is it possible.

ENDNOTES

1. 1 Corinthians 6:19-20 NLT
2. Hebrews 12:1-3 MSG
3. 1 Corinthians 9:24-27 NIV
4. Deuteronomy 30:19-20 NLT

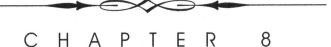

# UNPROTECTED

*"He will cover you with His feathers. He will shelter you with His wings. His faithful promises are your armor and protection."*

Psalm 91:4 NLT

F ear hit me. I had no idea where it came from, but I felt unprotected, like God would no longer help me on my journey. I was afraid He would not be there to remind me not to eat the things which would keep me on track. It was strange because I knew I had already dealt with this issue, and God and I had successfully eradicated the donut-eating monster.

One thing I have learned is when issues present themselves again, there is probably another area which needs to be examined. I no longer panic when God reveals an issue to me. I rejoice, because I know He's continuing to work on my behalf.

I know the exact beginning of some fears. Others are hidden in the recesses of my subconscious mind. They are like an emotional sound track which gets triggered at odd times. The evil one knows this and tries to bury the memory of what caused the fear while still keeping the door of fear open.

Once I understand a fear of some kind exists, I need only ask God to show me the first time I felt that kind of fear. When I know the root, God and I can easily thwart the evil one's effort. I am connected to a humongous God and the battle really does belong to Him. There happens to be a teeny, tiny little devil who is nothing compared to God. He is only powerful if I give him power.[1] Otherwise, all he can do is whisper lies in my ear, and remind me of who I am not. "There is no truth in him ... he is a liar and the father of lies."[2]

When God reveals the root source, breaking the emotional bondage is the next step. The deceiver[3] likes to disguise or bury the precipitating incident so I don't recognize it as being anything substantial. It's always the first time I felt the particular fear in some shape or form.

Such was the case with feeling unprotected. It was a door of fear open in my life. I had no idea where or how it got opened, I just knew it was open. When I asked God, He showed me the following incident. When He showed me, I remembered the situation, but didn't understand the connection until He revealed it.

## DRUNK IN THE DRIVEWAY

I was about 14. We had pulled up in the driveway of Grandma's two-story farmhouse. Pulled down farther in the drive was a car we didn't recognize.

There was a man in the car. His head was sort-of bobbling around. Then he rested it against the back of the seat like he was asleep.

I wanted my dad to go and see what was the matter with the man. He said we should go inside first.

My grandmother waited at the door anxiously wringing a dish towel between her hands.

"Ernie, I'm so glad you're here. I need you to go tell that man he needs to leave. Slim is gone to town, and the deputy can't be out here for two hours."

**Dad grew up poor, but not because his father didn't work.**

"Has he threatened you?"

"No. He hasn't gotten out of the car. I know who he is. He's a distant cousin, and he's a drunk. No telling what he'll do if he gets out of the car. I just want him off of the property."

"He has passed out. He won't hurt you. It could be bad news if we tried to wake him up. It's best he not drive if he's drunk. He might kill someone. We just need to let him sleep it off."

Because Dad grew up with an alcoholic father, he knew about drunks. He had told me that many Friday evenings after his father got paid, his dad would first go buy a bag of groceries, and then go to the local tavern. He'd walk the five miles home and come in without his bag of groceries, which contained all the food the family had for the next week.

Dad and his brothers would have to back-track to town to find the bag. Most times, my grandfather would have set it down somewhere as he climbed over a fence.

Dad grew up poor, but not because his father didn't work. His father was a hard worker, but he just drank away his earnings.

Dad never spoke ill of his father, but I knew his concern about confronting the drunk in the driveway came from real life knowledge. He didn't want to get up close and personal with a drunk man. He also knew once the man passed out he would stay that way for quite some time.

## GRANDMA'S RESPONSE

I could tell Grandma was not happy with Dad's solution. He had things he needed to do over on his farm, though. So, while the rest of my family went to the other farm about 10 miles away, I stayed to protect Grandma.

She was anxious and fidgety, looking out the window often until the sheriff's deputy arrived several hours later and carted the man off to jail.

I hadn't thought of this incident in years. I was only reminded of it when praying about issues of fear in my life and why I still felt unprotected.

The reason I felt unprotected was because on that occasion. I partnered with Grandma's fear. As a child I would have been fine had she not been so scared. By identifying Dad as the one who should have stayed to protect us, I had internalized Father God would not protect me in other ways. As I remembered the incident, the picture of Grandma and I being two little girls alone against a bad man came to my mind, and I felt the fear. It was as tangible as it had been when it happened.

I simply chose to forgive Dad for his absence even though he was a wonderful, godly man. Everything he did in that situation was good based on his knowledge of alcoholism. This was a rationalization of the adult part of me. Up until that time, the emotional part of me was still a little girl partnering with Grandma's anxiety.

Since my father had already passed away, this was not the type of forgiveness where I could go up to him and say, "I forgive you for not staying to protect us from the bad, drunk guy Grandma was scared of."

It is simply saying to Father God, "I choose to forgive my dad for not staying to protect us from the drunk man. I choose to forgive him for not understanding Grandma's fear. I choose to forgive him for leaving me there even though I would have been angry if I couldn't stay."

Then I renounced the lie Father God will not protect me from dangers. I renounced the lie He doesn't understand why I'm afraid, and He won't anticipate me being afraid. I renounced the lie Father God does not and will not watch out for me.

Finally, I asked, "Father God, what is Your truth?" I immediately heard, "I am with you always.[4] I will never leave you.[5] I will shelter you under the shadow of My wings.[6] I will cover you when you are afraid. You can trust in Me."[7]

## FORGIVING GRANDMA

I wasn't finished yet. There was another person I had to forgive. I had bonded with Grandma in a kind of soul-tie regarding the anxiety of feeling unprotected. Being the child in the situation I took on her feelings while at the same time trying to protect her.

I forgave her for unknowingly transferring this feeling to me. I broke the soul tie by giving back the fear to Grandma and taking back whatever she had unknowingly taken from me in the process. Before the incident I felt protected. Afterwards I felt vulnerable. So I took back the sense of protection.

In talking with Father God about this, I gave Him my anxiety, fear and feeling of not being protected. I asked, "What do You give me in exchange?"

Immediately, I sensed peace and calm fall over me. I also knew He spoke to my mind and said, "I give you My peace.[8] I am with you always.[9] You never need to be afraid. I am by your side."

## WHERE WERE YOU, JESUS?

As a child I'd always wondered where Jesus lived. I figured He lived with us because He was in our hearts. However, I just wanted to know where He resided. Problem was, our house was tiny. The room I shared with my sister was basically the end of a hallway. My brother's room used to be a back porch.

When I became an adult I knew the Holy Spirit, who is the Spirit of Christ, is the One who lives inside of me. Rational thoughts I have as an adult, however, do not answer the questions I had as a child. At times I felt Jesus didn't have my back. These were times like when Mom and I got into arguments or when she spanked me and I felt I had done nothing to deserve it.

Where were You, Jesus, during all the hard times in my life while I was growing up? I was an adult before I understood this was a question I could ask Jesus and He wouldn't think me crazy. I began to understand He longs to answer any questions which cause confusion, pain and doubt. So, I simply asked, "Where were You when I was growing up, Jesus?"

Immediately, I saw a vivid picture of Him engulfing our little white house with all of us safely inside. He did not have a room in our house. He was our house.

His very presence emanated from the corner of the living room where the old red chair sat, the one Dad had upholstered with a soft, black material. It was my father's prayer altar. Every evening at 10:30 p.m., he'd kneel in front of the chair to talk with Jesus after reading his Bible.

Jesus was taking loving care of me all those years. He would not interfere with my life, but He would hold me safely in His arms and watch over me and my family. He would answer Dad's heartfelt prayers for each of us, including my mother.

I firmly believe Jesus heard Dad's prayers and held us safe. It's why I'm still alive today. It's why I love Jesus with all my heart. My Dad's life of prayer and faith taught me that.

## WHERE IS JESUS TODAY?

Understanding where Jesus is still affects me profoundly. Recently, I woke up at three in the morning from a crazy dream. I was at an old house where we used to live. People were driving their cars up on our lawn, playing music, sitting on their cars, drinking, dancing, talking loudly and laughing uproariously. My husband and I were sitting on our front porch trying to have a quiet evening.

More people from the neighborhood began showing up, uninvited. At first, it was pleasant. Then, it turned nasty. One woman wanted to dig up my flower beds so she could have "good dirt" to plant her flowers. I nicely told her she could have any dirt in the yard, but not the dirt from my flower bed.

She started yelling at me, telling me I was selfish and calling me names. Others joined her rage. My husband and I looked at each other and quickly went inside locking all the doors and windows to protect our two children.

I panicked. I was afraid the crowd would break down the doors and storm into our house.

I woke up anxious. My mind shifted to the house we live in now. Were the doors and windows all locked? I began thinking of all the ways someone could get into the house if they wanted. I thought about going downstairs and making sure doors and windows were locked. I thought seriously about waking my husband.

**Logic, though, is never a component of panic.**

I got out of bed and began to think, "Why am I in a panic over a dream? Do I have a logical reason to be afraid?" I have never really experienced this kind of anxiety. Nothing in my dream was logical. Logic, though, is never a component of panic, which basically is fear.

I knew enough to hand these feelings to Jesus. In return, He gave me peace. However, I still didn't feel the presence of peace. I knew it was there, but it wasn't inside me yet. So, I asked, "Jesus, where are You in this house?"

His answer was quick. "This is a bigger house, but I've got this one, too. I'm bigger than your house.[10] I'm bigger than your panic. I'm bigger than your fear. I'm bigger than your problems.

All these years have I not taken care of you? I am this house, too. Wherever you are, I am already there."

I know now that Jesus is ever present with me. I do not have to be afraid.[11] Fear is simply false evidence appearing real. My dream was not real. The house was locked and safe. God's got this. More than that, God's got me. I don't have to be afraid.

## CLOSING THE DOOR OF FEAR

I know if I leave the door of fear open, fear will step in again. I must deal with fear as it arises and keep it out. Looking back, I now know I tried to protect myself by allowing extreme weight gain. Even though my rational mind wanted it gone, my emotional being wanted it present in order to feel protected.

The interesting thing is, weight gain does not and cannot protect me. When I am heavy, I can't run. I don't have the muscle mass I need, or the strength I need to protect myself. My immune system is weaker because of the unhealthy foods I consume. I am more susceptible to all kinds of diseases.

I was not protecting myself by gaining weight or becoming bigger than whoever might choose to harm me. Instead, I was leaving myself wide open for attack.

The enemy sets up lies and wants to use fear to lead me astray and cause my demise. He wants to limit what I can do for the Kingdom of God. He does not want fear erased. However, with God's help now I can identify what he's up to. I can erase the fear through prayer and forgiveness.

God promises to protect me. I'm grateful for Scripture verses which have been implanted in my heart. In times of despair His words come back to remind me that He's always here watching over me.

This was true recently when I was coming home from my exercise time. I was on the interstate, which I take nearly everyday. I was in the driving lane going less than the speed limit when I looked to my right, and a car was inches from my passenger side door apparently attempting to merge onto the highway.

**God, You must have something more for me to do here on earth because I should be dead right now. I just danced with a semi and lived to tell about it.**

As I swerved my small car to miss her, a semi passing on the other side caught my side view mirror. The next few moments were a blur as the air bags deployed, and I bounced off the semi not once, but twice.

Miraculously, I was able to get my car safely to the side of the busy interstate. The first words out of my mouth were, "God, You must have something more for me to do here on earth because I should be dead right now. I just danced with a semi and lived to tell about it."

My car was totaled, but I only had a scratch from the seat belt. I will never again doubt I have a squadron of guardian angels actively protecting me.

These are the verses which the Holy Spirit brought my mind and used to minister to me as I sat on the side of the interstate waiting for the myriad of emergency vehicles to arrive.

"What time I am afraid, I will trust in Thee."[12]

"There is no fear in love, but perfect love casts out fear."[13]

"Yea, though I walk through the valley of the shadow of death, I will fear no evil; for You are with me; Your rod and Your staff, they comfort me."[14]

"I sought the Lord, and He heard me, and delivered me from all my fears."[15]

"Fear not, for I am with you; be not dismayed, for I am your God. I will strengthen you. Yes, I will help you. I will uphold you with My righteous right hand."[16]

"For God has not given us a spirit of fear, but of power and of love and of a sound mind."[17]

Psalm 91 has long been a favorite chapter in the Bible. These are some of my special verses of comfort and assurance. "Those who live in the shelter of the Most High will find rest in the shadow of the Almighty. This I declare about the Lord: 'He alone is my refuge, my place of safety; He is my God, and I trust Him.

**"He will cover you with His feathers. He will shelter you with His wings. His faithful promises are your armor and protection."**

"He will cover you with His feathers. He will shelter you with His wings. His faithful promises are your armor and protection. For He will order His angels to protect you wherever you go. They will hold you up with their hands so you won't even hurt your foot on a stone.'"[18]

Feeling protected was so important on my journey. Just as important, though, was understanding my failures. I have had a lot of them, but I had no idea greed was one of them.

## ENDNOTES

1.  1 John 4:4 NKJV, James 4:7 NKJV
2.  John 8:44 NIV
3.  Revelation 12:9 NKJV
4.  Matthew 28:20 NKJV
5.  Hebrews 13:5 NKJV
6.  Psalm 17:8, 36:7, 57:1, 63:7 NKJV
7.  Psalm 91:4 NLT
8.  John 14:27 NIV
9.  Hebrews 13:5 NIV
10.  Isaiah 66:1 NIV
11.  Psalm 91:4-5 NLT
12.  Psalm 56:3 KJV
13.  1 John 4:18 NKJV
14.  Psalm 23:4 NKJV
15.  Psalm 34:4 NKJV
16.  Isaiah 41:10 NKJV
17.  2 Timothy 1:7 NKJV
18.  Psalm 91:1-2, 4, 11-12 NLT

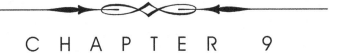

# GREED

*"We are God's poetry, a recreated people who will fulfill the destiny He has given each of us, for we are joined to Jesus, the Anointed One. Even before we were born, God planned in advance our destiny and the good works we would do to fulfill it."*

Ephesians 2:10 TPT

When I was seven years old, I was eating out of the devil's hands, literally. It happened at the end of our family's Friday night ritual of grocery shopping. Dad would always give my brother and I a dime for being good. We'd buy penny candy with it.

This night we'd been good, but at the checkout counter Dad told us he didn't have extra money to give us. I was mad. I had earned my candy. I wanted my candy. I could taste the sweet, buttery flavor of my favorite caramels.

I knew throwing a temper tantrum wouldn't work. So I just slipped some penny candies in my coat pocket. It was greed, pure and simple. I wanted it. I took it.

When Dad learned what I had done, he took me back to the store and told the manager I had something to tell him. So, I confessed. Then, Dad paid my debt.

When we were walking out of the store I saw the tear in Dad's eyes. I realized that I am the sinner the preacher hollers about. Later that day, I confessed my sin to Jesus, and invited Him into my heart.

God used this difficult situation to bring about a saving change in my life.[1] I repented of stealing candy from the store. I knew stealing was wrong because the Bible clearly says not to steal.[2] What I didn't realize then was how stealing is effectively greed. I had been greedy in this situation. I wanted candy, and I was going to have it. It didn't matter if I had money or not.

## GREEDY

Greed says, "I will have this because I want it even if I can't afford it." It is usually used in the context of material possessions. At its core, the excessive want of anything is greed, especially when one consumes more than their share.

As a seven-year-old, my greed was lust for what I desired. It began to build into a gluttonous attitude of always wanting more of what filled a void in my life. Finally, it pushed me to want more than my portion of any food.

It went beyond childhood to when I was a teenager squandering money on eating out. This was money I made and was supposed to be saving for college.

It continued after I graduated college and went to work at my first full-time job. I spent whatever I wanted, whenever I wanted. I went out to eat all the time. I just put it all on that newly acquired wonder called the credit card.

This only became worse when, as a young family, we were struggling financially. I would put groceries on the credit card. I mean, my kids have to eat, right? However, they needed healthy meals, not the bags of junk food I'd bring into the house only for it to disappear as quickly as it came in.

My kids didn't eat that much. My husband rarely touched the chips, cookies and candy. Guess who that left? In essence, I was stealing food from my family. I was using money I didn't have to purchase food I didn't need. If I needed to food on credit, in the very least, it should have been healthy food.

It was clear to me. This all began because I dealt with the sin of stealing, but I never dealt with the sin of the greed of wanting candy any way I could get it. I knew the Bible said, do not steal. I also knew it didn't say, do not eat candy.

It's still amazing to me how something which happened when I was seven could affect my emotional core as a mature adult. I didn't see the issue until I had lost the bulk of my weight.

## PRESENTING ISSUE

The presenting issue, though, was something different. I had been struggling with what I described to myself as a poverty mentality. It had to do with money and feeling like it's not right to make money from ministry. I knew this was not true, but it was still strong within me. When I would think about charging for something, I just couldn't bring myself to do it, and I didn't know why.

I always thought I had to have a secular job to support what I did. I was struggling to place a price on the various types of coaching I do, all of which are based on spiritual principles. In my mind, it was clearly ministry, and I wasn't sure if I could or should seek to make money from helping people.

## THE NOTHING WALL

I understood there was a barrier or a wall between God and I in regard to this. It was a different kind of wall, though, one which I had never encountered personally. I closed my eyes and asked God to show me the wall. It was white, almost like a nothing wall.

"Ask Jesus to remove the wall," the coach helping me said. It was a very matter-of-fact statement. So, I closed my eyes and did what she said to do. I saw the wall, and I saw Jesus. He simply waved His hand from the right to the left and the nothing wall drew back like a curtain.

Behind it was Father God standing looking at me.

She quietly asked, "What do you see?"

"I see Father God."

"Do you feel comfortable talking with Him?"

"Yes."

I had no thought the wall was related to the grocery store incident. That was the last thing on my mind. The coach knew, though. She said, "Ask Him, 'Father God, where were You that day in the market?'"

I did, and then answered, "He was in my heart."

Again she prompted me to ask, "Father God, what do You want me to know about that day?"

I answered, "God wants me to know my father was protecting me."

At her prompt, I asked, "Father God, what was Dad protecting me from?"

I added when I heard the answer. "Greed. He was protecting me from being greedy."

Then, I asked, "Father God, what lie am I believing about greed?"

He told me the lie I was believing was I couldn't have what I want.

> I was believing God wouldn't provide for me in my ministry calling.

After a pause she led me to forgive my dad for not letting me have what I wanted that day. I forgave him for saying, "No," to me and for not having enough money for what I wanted.

Then I asked, "Father God, is there a lie I am believing?" Immediately I sensed He said, "Yes." So I asked, "What lie am I believing?"

The realization came. I was believing God wouldn't provide for me in my ministry calling. I was believing He wouldn't give me what I wanted because He didn't have enough. I was believing He would make me work at something I simply tolerate in order to do what I love doing which is helping people find freedom.

In every failure, God teaches me a lesson. That day I learned there are perimeters around what I can and can't have. When I try to get what I want my way, instead of doing what God has told me or shown me to do, it never ends well.

The lesson went beyond finances. I saw how much it related to food, also. For the last several years I had been doing what God told me to do regarding what and how much I eat and how I move. I'd seen great results by following Him.

Looking back over my life, though, I saw how I violated the perimeters of what I can and can't have. I did this by buying food I wanted on credit when we didn't have money for it.

This situation was in my past. We had recovered from it financially, and were managing our money well. Still, I knew I needed to give this failure to God. When I handed it to Him, He gave me forgiveness.

It felt like a weight had been lifted. I had been carrying around a bag full of failure. It was always in the back of my mind, in the subscript of things playing across my inner big screen. When I asked and God forgave my greed and bad choices, it felt like the entire universe exhaled with my sigh of relief.

## MORE GREED

In the midst of not believing God would provide my needs and the needs of my family if I were doing ministry full-time, I realized there was another type of greed.

This type of greed was a more grown-up kind, which said, "God, I don't think You will provide enough money for us to live like we have been living, so I'll keep doing it myself if You don't mind."

When my coach asked me what I feared about letting go of my job, I immediately responded, "That we will be destitute on the street, and God will not provide at the level we are currently living. I want provision in a way where all the bills are paid and finances are not a worry. Will You do that, God?"

I heard His voice clearly answer, "I have provided all this time. I will continue to provide. If I have called you to do something, I will provide for you."[3]

## UNDERSTANDING PROVISION

Finally, I broke off the lie Dad did not provide for me that day in the grocery store, and that Father God will not provide. Then I asked Him, "What is Your truth?"

The truth is I was greedy when I was seven and many times throughout the years. My greed made me feel I could never have what I wanted, and what I felt I had earned. I handed this greed to God and He gave me forgiveness. The God of the Universe forgave my greed without hesitation. It was an amazingly freeing feeling.

One final step, though, was very necessary. I realized I had taken on the role of provider for my family. This was never supposed to be mine. Ultimately, God is our family's provider. I thought I had a better plan.

I handed the role of provider back to Father God. He gave me destiny and purpose in exchange. He gave me what has become one of my favorite verses.

"We have become His poetry, a recreated people that will fulfill the destiny He has given each of us, for we are joined to Jesus, the Anointed One. Even before we were born, God planned in advance our destiny and the good works we would do to fulfill it."[4]

Like the song says, "He's a good, good father. It is who He is. It's who He is. And I am loved by Him. It's who I am. It's who I am."[5] What I need to do is step into the truth of that.

If He loves me, I should love and take care of myself. I need to understand God does not want me to work long hours and further damage my body with stress and lack of sleep.

## God wants me healthy—body, soul and spirit.

God wants me healthy—body, soul and spirit. I had learned this regarding the wrong habits which led me to gain weight. Now, I was eating correctly and exercising six days a week. However, in the area of rest and relaxation, I was sadly lacking.

God understands my limits even when I don't. He is my Father, my provider. I asked Him to show me how to make time for rest and relaxation. The feeling I have to work hard at a regular job in order to do the ministry I love is a lie.

I'll admit I am a work in progress. I recognize the lie. I realize the truth. I know the action steps I need to do to make it happen. I've put in place a plan to get to bed earlier and find times of refreshing, get-aways with my husband or good friends. I'm asking God to lead me step-by-step in this area and remind me when I'm not following His directions.

Every failure I have had has been an opportunity to allow God to remove another lie so I don't return to the sickening depths of super morbid obesity.

I know if I'm spending time with Him, reading His Word, listening to His instructions, He will reveal any lies I am believing and make the truth plain.

When I come to Christ, He forgives my failures—past, present and future. "Through the blood of his Son, we are set free from our sins. God forgives our failures because of His overflowing kindness. He poured

**The weight is gone for good, never to return as long as I am following Him.**

out His kindness by giving us every kind of wisdom and insight."[6]

I need not be worried about these failures or sins returning. He says He has removed my sins as far as the east is from the west.[7] He will have compassion on me. He will trample my sins under His feet and throw them into the depths of the ocean.[8]

I feel confident that thanks to God helping me overcome significant barriers, the weight is gone, never to return as long as I am following Him. Still, I must always be aware there is an enemy of my soul. He is the master manipulator. He will steal my victory if I allow him even an inch of territory.

## ENDNOTES

1. Romans 8:28 NIV
2. Exodus 20:15 NIV
3. 1 Thessalonians 5:24 NIV
4. Ephesians 2:10 TPT
5. Barrett, Pat, and Tony Brown. Good, Good Father. Housefires. Rec. 9 Sept. 2014. 2014. Web.
6. Ephesians 1:7-8 GW
7. Psalm 103:12 NLT
8. Micah 7:19 NLT

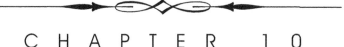

CHAPTER 10

# DECEPTION

*"You saw me before I was born. Every day of my life was recorded in Your book. Every moment was laid out before a single day had passed."*

Psalm 139:16 NLT

I know what hell is like. Hell is when I find myself weighing 430 pounds and know I have put myself there. Hell is wanting to stop eating, trying to stop, but feeling powerless to do so.

Hell is feeling like I am standing on a railroad track watching a locomotive speeding towards me, but feeling too paralyzed to move, and not knowing why.

Hell is realizing I must do something to stop eating, but like an airplane on autopilot I keep going full speed knowing what the end result will be.

Hell is not being able to enjoy life because all I can think about is what I am currently consuming and how I can get some more, much like a drug addict awaiting the next hit.

Hell is wanting to be normal, but hopeless that normal can ever happen to me.

Hell is having the foods I love turn on me, and with angry claws and fangs begin to devour me.

Hell is denying all of this is going on while trying to smile and live an ordinary life when inside I feel dead. Except, of course, when I eat something decadent and then, the cycle starts over again.

Hell is knowing all of this is my fault, but not knowing how to do what I know to do.

Hell is understanding God has a better plan for my life, and knowing I have willfully ignored and thwarted it.

Hell is living mired in lies and half-truths, which have me bound and gagged.

Hell is living for the next time I can gorge myself with rich, sugary breads and foods.

Hell is knowing I breathe for one reason and one reason only—the next time I can eat.

## LIVING HELL

I don't like hell. I have been there and lived there for over half of my life. I am determined never to return. However, I also well know while I was there Satan, the father of lies,[1] the master deceiver,[2] had me convinced where I was living was heaven.

I saw all the things I loved to eat as heavenly. Some of them were even packaged with words like heavenly cakes, delightful treats, good bars and too good to be true candy. When someone would say, "Think of the most heavenly thing on earth," my mind would not go to a pastor or some great missionary or person I knew who was godly. No, my mind went to something delicious my grandmother and all the wonderful great aunts made while I was growing up.

Being in heaven would be like being at a great feast, which lasted continually. It would be eating anything and everything I wanted. This was my idea of heaven. It had nothing to do with the presence of God, and everything with the presence of my favorite foods.

I had definitely been deceived.

## THE DECEIVER

A person who deceives is one who misleads by a false appearance or statement. Isn't it interesting Satan can appear as an angel of light[3]? Many times in Scripture we experience him misleading people by saying something which isn't true.

The first deception was the serpent deceiving Eve. It was paradise in the Garden of Eden, but death entered the world that day when Eve gave into the devil's temptation to eat food she knew God didn't want her to eat.

Why didn't He want her to eat this specific food? Because He knew it would eventually lead to her death. He even told her this very thing. Yet evil argued against it saying, "You're crazy. You won't die if you eat this food, which looks beautiful[4] and delicious. You'll just get smarter and wiser like God is.[5] This is God's food, but you deserve it too. Go ahead, eat it."

It was a dual trap. Eat the food because of its looks and taste. Eat the food because of how it will make you feel.

Many times I have done the same thing. The food was arranged in a delectable presentation. Maybe I saw it on a commercial and I salivated seeing how yummy it looked. So,

I drove to the tree, in this case probably a fast food restaurant, and put myself in harm's way.

## THE DECEIVED

When I walked in, I could smell the special concoction they had advertised. The actual food itself looked juicy and delicious. I could taste it. By this time, there was no turning back. I had to have it. Oh, and the fact the commercial said it was made from some healthy ingredient or another supposedly making it good for me, just sealed the deal.

Maybe this is not an accurate depiction of the first temptation, but to me Eve's fall was all about the food, and not really too much about what it might do for her. She just needed an excuse to try the one food God had made off limits to her.

The devil is a deceiver who turns something, which looks good, into something, which leads to death, even though it may be a while coming.

Although she had other consequences because of eating of the forbidden tree, I'm sure Eve never thought a seemingly casual food choice would impact future generations, which would include not only herself, Adam and her twin sons, but all of humankind.

She didn't have the insight to comprehend when God says, "Don't," He means, "Don't." He doesn't limit individuals because He's mean. He gives directions for people to be able to live life to the fullest, in abundance, because He knows what's best.

# THE DECEPTION

Part of the deception I bought into was believing food was just food. God made food for us to eat and enjoy, so I could eat whatever I wanted whenever I wanted.

I justified this from Scripture, where Jesus is quoted as declaring all foods clean to eat. "'Don't you see that nothing that enters a person from the outside can defile them? For it doesn't go into their heart, but into their stomach and then out of the body.'

"In saying this, Jesus declared all foods clean. He went on: 'What comes out of a person is what defiles them. For it is from within, out of a person's heart, that evil thoughts come—sexual immorality, theft, murder, adultery, greed, malice, deceit, lewdness, envy, slander, arrogance and folly. All these evils come from inside and defile a person.'"[6]

I twisted this to say, "Jesus said I can eat whatever I want." The truth is, it is permissible for me to eat anything, except if it masters or controls me. "All things are lawful for me, but not all things are profitable. All things are lawful for me, but I will not be mastered by anything."[7]

## SOURCE OF MY DECEPTION

I had been deceived, and I couldn't blame anyone but myself. I wanted certain foods. I thought I had to have them to survive. Surely Jesus understood eating good food. He was human. He ate meals. However, He did not allow what He ate to be something which controlled His heart, the seat of His emotions.

I did, though. I thought I had to have comfort foods to make me halfway normal. It seemed to be the only way I could calm any frustration, anger or what I considered the ugly emotions.

> It seemed to be the only way I could calm any frustration, anger or what I considered the ugly emotions.

One incident that really stands out in my mind happened when I was a teenager, around 13. It was a summer afternoon, and I was in my room reading. My brother and sister were outside playing, but I had sneaked back in to have some quiet time.

My mother was in the living room. Belva, a neighbor, came over. She and Mom began talking. I wasn't really listening, but in our small house it was impossible not to hear. The air return grate between my closet and the living room carried any sound directly into my room.

"I sure do love your daughter," Belva said. "Teresa's always so nice and sweet with all the kids." I blushed. I liked Belva. She was fun.

However, the next statement wasn't fun at all.

"She certainly isn't that way here at home," Mom said. "She's rude, hateful and mean."

"Really? I can't imagine that. She's great at my house."

"You seem to be talking about a different person. She's not so great here."

I was floored. My mother thought I was rude, hateful and mean. What she said made me feel broken and sad. What a horrible Christian I was. Repenting of my failure wasn't really on my list of things to do right then. All I wanted was to find something to eat to make me feel better, but Mom and Belva were still in the living room. I couldn't sneak into the kitchen.

So, I began to think about my last interaction with Belva. We had played cards, laughed and talked. I really loved just having a good time with her. Then I thought about the last interaction with Mom. She had been upset about something. She had spoken loudly and, of course, I had screamed back.

I watched the argument replay in slow motion across my mind. I realized she had an emotional instability, and by yelling back at her, even though what she said made me angry, all I did was escalate the problem.

I decided right then, I'd be as nice at home as I was other places. I wouldn't yell at my mother no matter how angry it made me.

In a few minutes, Belva asked Mom to come over to her house to look at something. As soon as I heard the door close, I went in search of the bag of caramels I knew Mom kept hidden in her room. I ate as many as I dared. I needed to get rid of the anger I felt at Mom's words, even though they were true.

> Every time I wanted to yell, I heard my mother's voice saying, "She's rude, hateful and mean."

I was nice after that. It was hard not to be. Every time I wanted to yell, I heard my mother's voice saying, "She's rude, hateful and mean." I'd force myself to keep calm and not say something I regretted. Then, I had to put something in my mouth to keep from screaming, preferably something sweet. I thought I was getting rid of the frustration building inside, instead I was stuffing it down further and further with food.

## FORGIVING DECEPTION

A deception is a lie, pure and simple. The lie I believed was food can relieve anger and frustration. It was sort-of a secret belief. I knew, even after losing over 260 pounds, I needed to confront this head on.

It definitely called for me to forgive Mom once again, even though I knew I was really at fault. After all, I was the one screaming at her. I was responsible for that action. However, I was still an adolescent who felt she had to stuff her anger because of something her mother said.

I began simply. "I choose to forgive Mom for saying I was rude, hateful and mean. I choose to forgive her for making me feel I couldn't express my emotions. I choose to forgive her for setting up the situation where I began to stuff my emotions with food instead of finding a better method of dealing with them. I choose to forgive Mom for not liking me when I was angry and for making me feel anger is a bad thing to express."

I continued, "I renounce the lie You, Holy Spirit, believe I am rude, hateful and mean. I renounce the lie You don't want me to express my emotions, instead I must hide them. I renounce the lie You don't like me when I'm emotional, and You only like me when I'm sweet and quiet. I renounce the lie You think it is better when I stuff my emotions."

Then, I asked Holy Spirit, "What is Your truth? His words soothed my soul as only the Comforter can.

He said, "I created you. I love the unique and wonderful woman you are. I loved you before you were born.[8] I saw your specialness then. I created you for a purpose. Do not let anger or stuffing anger thwart your destiny in Me."[9]

Afterwards, I knew I needed to do something else. I handed my anger to the Holy Spirit. I handed the foods I used to stop any anger or frustration to Him.

In the place of those things He said, "I give you peace, My peace,[10] the only truly real peace, a commodity, which is in such short supply today. I need you to receive My peace. I need you to be a bearer of My peace. Will you receive My peace? Will you share it with others?"

## DEEPER TRUTH

The moment I said, "Yes," I began to realize a deep truth. God gives us the opposite of what the devil wants us to believe. The devil uses our own desires to set up deception in us. I thought food was an acceptable thing to live for. The devil agreed because living to eat meant I was not living for God.

I was living for the next thing to give me pleasure. Ungodly pleasure is anything I put above God. For me, it was the foods I craved and allowed to master me. Just the subtle thought these foods were heavenly made it acceptable for me to continue eating them anytime I wanted and as much as I wanted.

When I gained an ungodly amount of weight, and God nudged me to show me the right course of action, I stubbornly stood my ground. This was my food, and I wanted it. It's the one thing I can have. The church says I can't drink, do drugs, lie, steal, have sex outside of marriage, but I can eat, so there.

This idea that food was an acceptable way to overcome any pain or emotional outburst is the devil's perversion of what helps me live.

I cannot live without food. However, I can live without certain foods, especially if when I start eating them I can't seem to stop.

> I no longer live to eat. Instead, I eat to live. When I find certain foods are controlling me, I stop eating them. I only want to be controlled by God.

I've learned for me it's better to not eat foods made with sugar, flour and gluten. If I stay away from them, I can eat healthy. If I start to eat the other foods, I have knowingly put myself back in prison.

With the help of Holy Spirit dropping real truth into my being, I have done a complete turn-around. I no longer live to eat. Instead, I eat to live. When I find certain foods are controlling me, I stop eating them. I only want to be controlled by God.

One way leads to death, maybe a slow death, but an earlier death than necessary, nonetheless. The other way leads to life. I will choose life.[11]

I am no longer deceived. I know the truth now. To deny it would mean I am rejecting my Savior. It might not mean I would be barred from heaven, but it would mean I would no longer hear His voice, be in His presence or fulfill the destiny[12] He has for me.

That would be hell.

134

My mother finally chose to pursue God with everything within her. In what I consider to be a miraculous turn of events, her darkness was turned to light. She became my inspiration. It's a story I love to tell because it propelled me forward on my journey.

## ENDNOTES

1.   John 8:44 TLB

2.   Revelation 20:3 AMP

3.   2 Corinthians 11:14 AMP

4.   Genesis 3:6 NLT

5.   Genesis 3:4-5 AMP

6.   Mark 7:18-23 NIV

7.   1 Corinthians 6:12 NASB

8.   Psalm 139: 13-16 NLT

9.   Ephesians 2:10 TPT

10.  John 14:27 NLT, Philippians 4:7 NLT

11.  Deuteronomy 30:19-20 NLT

12.  Ephesians 2:10 TPT

SWEET FREEDOM

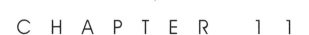

CHAPTER 11

# UNANSWERED PRAYER

*"I sought the Lord, and He heard me, and
delivered me from all my fears."*

Psalm 34:4 NKJV

M y friend, if you're listening right now to me, this is the moment you can be free. This very same Jesus is right here today. Release your faith and touch Him, then believe me when I say, "Something good is going to happen to you, happen to you this very day. Something good is going to happen to you, Jesus of Nazareth is passing this way."[1]

Watching the Oral Roberts Show became a highlight of the week for me. I sat as close to the TV screen as possible, primarily because I didn't want to miss the time when Bro. Roberts turned to the TV screen and spoke directly to me.

"Those of you watching by television can receive your miracle today," he said. "Just lay your hands on the TV screen while I pray." Those might not have been the exact words, but they were close. Then he'd pray for my personal miracle.

I just knew God could hear him better than me. Every week I saw people walk across the stage and receive healing, shouting praises to God. I would pray, believing my mother would be healed of whatever illness was besetting her, the one which made her different from other mothers.

As early as I can remember, my mother's healing topped every prayer list I made. It was the subject of every spoken and unspoken prayer request in church and Sunday School, the thing my grandmother and I prayed for each time I spent the weekend with her and what Dad prayed for every night.

With that much prayer going up on her behalf, I knew one day God might just get fed up with hearing her name on everyone's prayer list and grant the request just so we'd all move on to something else.

## WHAT'S WRONG WITH MOM?

My mother's illness was characterized by extremes—highs, lows, anger, sadness, happiness and complete withdrawal. She saw a psychiatrist weekly and took medications.

As I was growing up, though, I had no concept of what my mother was going through. As a kid, all I knew was my mother was different from the other mothers. She did not like crowds or big events so she never came to anything I was involved in at school. I can't remember her coming to a parent-teacher conference, a school play, a band concert or an awards assembly even though I was part of all of those.

My friends' mothers came and congratulated me for everything I did, but my mother was conspicuously absent, at least it was conspicuous to me. I longed for her to come, just once. I prayed for her to come, but she never did.

My father made sure we never missed a church service. We were there Sunday morning, Sunday night, Wednesday night and Friday night, not to mention numerous revival services. Sometimes Mom came, and sometimes she didn't. A lot depended on if she was "sick" or not.

She loved Jesus, it was just that crowds made her anxious or as she would say, "Crowds makes me nervous." She always felt she didn't measure up. Her quest for perfection was unrealistic, but always in front of her.

Many times she would say she felt she wasn't good enough to be in church. She should play the piano. She should lead music. She should teach Sunday School. She should go to women's meetings. The things she felt she should be and do would defeat and shame her to the point she could not bring herself to face a group of people she had decided were judging her.

## UNDERSTANDING SHAME

Years later, I would understand some of what she felt. When I weighed 430 pounds, and even before I got to that point, I had a habit of walking into church and immediately surveying the crowd to see if I was the largest one there.

My feeling of inadequacy was not predicated by anyone who looked down on me. It was totally and completely based on the shame and guilt I felt for allowing myself to get into the predicament I was in. Still, to deny its existence would be false. It was there. I couldn't shake it.

The same was true for Mom. Others knew she had an illness. Not everyone knew what it was, or even if it was emotionally or psychologically based. My father was a quiet man. He didn't share prayer requests with everyone. He just prayed fervently.

Mom was sure everyone thought she was crazy and was judging her because of her issues. She preferred to stay away. That way she didn't have to wonder what others might be thinking.

What she didn't understand was many were praying for her even though they might not know the exact issue she was facing. They knew she was sick and that was enough information for them to pray.

# FEAR

There were several years when Mom did not even want Dad to leave her on Sunday morning to go to church. During that time, he sent my brother and I to the church across the street from our house. At the time, Dad knew the pastor there. He knew he would give us the Word even though it wasn't my father's chosen denomination.

It became my church. I made friends there and was well taken care of by several adopted mothers. One such lady was Betty. She lived in the neighborhood and knew the situation with my mother. She was a prayer warrior. Every time I saw her, she always told me she was praying for my mother.

It felt good to know Mom was on someone else's prayer list besides mine and my family's. It's sort-of required to pray when someone in your family has a great need. To know Betty also prayed helped me in a way I can't really explain. She didn't have to pray for Mom, but she did.

My prayers for Mom became more desperate as it drew closer to the time for me to leave for college. As far as I could tell, my brother and sister escaped a lot of the irrational behavior. I always encouraged them to go outside and play while I stayed inside. I really was more of an indoors person. Still, I tried to protect them until Dad got home.

I didn't know what would happen, though, when I left home. Would my brother and sister be targeted?

Writing prayer requests to Oral Roberts became something I regularly did. Though I never heard back personally from Oral, from time to time someone on his staff would send a form letter. Inside it would be another envelope and form to send back more prayer requests.

Many times, when I came home from school, Mom would be sitting in a near catatonic state in her chair in the living room. Each day, though, the mail would be on the side table by the door.

## MOM'S PRAYER REQUEST

One day I looked to see if I had any mail. I saw what I thought was a letter from Oral Roberts. I tore it open and saw my mother's handwriting. She had sent a prayer request to the organization asking for prayer.

What she wrote, made the color drain from my face. "Many times I feel like killing myself and my three children just to take them out of all the misery there is in this world. Please pray for me."

There she sat, just a few feet from me. She was staring as if she was seeing right through me. If she saw me read the letter, she made no indication. Did she want me to read it? Is that why she put it in the envelope which had my name on the return address?

## NOW WHAT?

In a month I was graduating from high school. At the end of the summer, I was bound for college. Scholarships were in place. My dorm room was ready. I would be fulfilling my dream to get a degree in journalism with a Christian emphasis.

Now what? I knew my mother was unstable, but I never considered her a threat. I was not worried about myself. In the last few years I knew I had become much stronger than her. I was concerned about protecting my brother and sister. I was also concerned about who would protect my mom from herself when I was 400 miles away.

Should I put college off until next year? I was prepared to go now, though. Postponing a dream I knew God had placed inside me did not seem like the answer either.

Mom was becoming increasingly unwilling to go anywhere. When Dad got home, he and I did the grocery shopping. I told him what I found. We cried and he promised me he would make sure all was OK at home.

"Your brother is old enough to take care of himself, and I will work it out so one of the neighbors looks out for your sister until I get home. She's got plenty of friends she hangs out with. I'll let their mothers know. God will protect them."

"But what can I do?" I said.

"First, you can pray. Never stop doing that. God always hears heartfelt prayers. Pray for your mother. She is an adult. Only God can keep her from doing something to herself, but I will make sure she doesn't have the means.

"Second, you can go to college. That's your job right now. I promise God and I will take care of things here."

A summer job at a local newspaper occupied the rest of my time at home. My prayer life seemed to take on an increased fervor, but it also became rather repetitive and boring. I saw no indication my prayers ever really reached beyond the ceiling.

I didn't know if God just didn't listen, or if He chose to ignore me. Although she did come to my high school graduation, it seemed Mom was getting worse rather than better. Frustration reigned, and pretty soon my prayers on behalf of my mother stopped altogether. They seemed fruitless. I felt God didn't care.

## BETTY'S PRAYERS

In addition to going to my church and living in my neighborhood, Betty also worked at the newspaper. At the end of the summer before I left for college, she caught me leaving work. I'd had a bad day and didn't want to see her. I didn't want to hear she was praying for my mother. I just couldn't stand to hear it one more time. I tried turning and going the other way.

"Teresa, when are you leaving for school?" she said smiling and giving me a hug.

I leaned into, but didn't return the hug. "This is my last day, thank God."

"I just want you to know, I'm praying for your momma."

I couldn't help it. I furrowed my brow and turned to face her. Even the lines of wisdom etched in her face and her smiling eyes couldn't deter me.

"Don't pray for her. God isn't going to answer. I've prayed for her for 18 years, and I've had no indication He has heard me once. There's no reason to pray. Don't waste your breath. My mother is a hopeless cause."

Fury rising inside, I stalked out the door. I could almost hear her as she mentally added me to her prayer list.

## THE PHONE CALL

College started for me. Though I vowed not to pray for Mom, she found her way to the top of my prayer list again. On my frequent calls home, I talked with my brother and sister who told me all about their friends. I would also talk to my mother, but I could tell her mood swings varied widely. Dad just sounded tired.

The astounding call from Mom came early in November.

"Teresa, are you sitting down," she said in a calm voice.

"What's up, Mom?"

"God healed me."

"What?" I wasn't sure I heard right.

"God healed me," she repeated with enthusiasm in her voice.

I'm not sure I said anything after that. Over the next few minutes she and Dad told me an incredible story.

Mom had gotten so bad she would not leave the house at all. She wouldn't go to church, the store, even to a friend's house. In the midst of this, a woman from the church in Jefferson City where Mom and Dad attended more than 15 years before called Mom out of the blue.

"There is a Full Gospel Businessmen's Fellowship Meeting in Columbia tonight," Yvonne said. "I'll be at your house by 6:30 p.m. to pick you up."

Miraculously, Mom agreed to go even though it had been months since she had been anywhere. Apparently Dad and my sister went as well, though I don't remember that part of the story. My sister was 10 or 11 at the time. She barely remembers the meeting. I remember vividly what Mom told me.

At the meeting, the evangelist spoke about emotional illness. After the message, he said, "There are three people here tonight whom God is going to touch. I want you to stand."

## GOD'S PLAN FOR FREEDOM

My anxiety-ridden, depressed, agoraphobic mother stood, along with two other people. He spoke individually to each one giving them God's plan for their freedom.

Mom was talking nonstop. I was standing in my dorm room with my mouth hanging open.

"When he got to me, the preacher said, 'God is going to touch you today and start you on your healing journey. You have been trying to fit the Bible into your life. You need to fit your life into the Bible. Don't look for passages in the Scripture to justify what you want to do. Do what the Bible tells you to do.'"

"What did you think of what he said?"

"As soon as he spoke those words, I knew they were for me. I knew I had been doing that. How did he know I'd search the Bible to justify what I wanted to do? It's not going to be easy, but at least now I have a plan of action, and I know now God has the power to help me get well."

"What are you going to do?"

"I'm going to hang on to Jesus just as tight as I can."

## HOLDING ON TO JESUS

So, she began her journey, tapping into the Word of God and hanging on to the very presence of Jesus in her life. She joined Dad for prayer times and Bible reading every morning and night. She focused on others instead of herself.

It was a long process and took years for her to step into her transformation, but eventually she became a loving and caring wife, mother and grandmother.

I had all but given up hope God could help my mother. I began to believe He couldn't answer the specific prayers I prayed. I started to believe my mother's struggles were bigger than God. Mom and God showed me differently.

I saw Jesus work in her life, and I saw her let Him. Still, I never wanted to have problems like her. I never wanted to act like what I thought was crazy or insane.

Fast forward to when I weighted 430 pounds and had a time limit of five years to live as declared by a doctor. I was eating anything and everything I could. I was acting like a crazy person.

There was only one other person I knew who had overcome something, which I felt was bigger than God. That person was my mother. I was going to have to give up sugar, the thing I craved constantly, the thing which kept me bound in a tomb of death, the thing which loomed like a monumental giant in my life, even bigger than my concept of God.

Because of my mother's phone call all those years ago, I knew beyond a shadow of a doubt that God had the power to help me overcome my monumental problem.

I spent all my life trying not to be like my mother and yet, right then I wanted nothing more than to be just like the woman I knew had overcome her emotional illness by the power of God. I began walking out my journey holding tight to Jesus. In the process I gave Him more than 260 of my unwanted pounds.

## DELIGHTING IN THE RIGHT THING

One of my mother's favorite verses summarizes how she turned her life around. "I sought the Lord, and He heard me, and delivered me from all my fears."[2] She knew only God could deliver her. She clung to that promise. She had to stop focusing on herself and focus on God. This was what the evangelist had told her.

It's the answer I am beginning to understand more and more each day. When I seek Him, my problems diminish. I can't help but surrender everything I'm afraid I can't live without to the One I never want to be without.

Another of her favorite verses says, "Delight yourself also in the Lord and He shall give you the desires of your heart."[3] He has become my delight and the real desire of my heart. I want nothing to stand in my way of following after Him.

## WALKING OUT HER JOURNEY

I am forever indebted to my mother who walked out her journey in front of me. She was a living demonstration that the power of God can and does transform lives.

I am overwhelmed by a God who cares so much about me He would walk with me through the hell of my life into the freedom[4] only He can bring.[5] He can change[6] me when I let Him.

By Thanksgiving, my mother was a different person. She started a journey the day the evangelist prayed for her and continued until the day she died in 1992. Though she still had some difficulties, each day got better.

The next time I saw Betty, I threw my arms around her and hugged her for a long time. I apologized for my insolent attitude, and thanked her for never giving up praying for my mother.

"I serve a God who always answers prayer," she said. "My job is to keep praying and have just a little more faith each day."

God gets all the glory for Mom's healing. What doctors, medications, outpatient clinics and mental hospitals couldn't do, God could and did. He did it in His time and in His way. It was His agenda completely.

There is a difference between a preacher telling me God has power to help me overcome, and when I see it lived out in another's life. My mother's life demonstrates one thing—God has power to change stuck lives.

When my grandpa would get the tractor stuck in the mud, he'd borrow teams of horses from neighboring farms to pull out what I thought of as the toughest piece of machinery on earth.

As powerful as the tractor was, it couldn't pull itself out when mired in mud up to the wheel hubs. He needed a power greater than what he had available to do the job. I would watch the horses work their magic as they slowly, but steadily pulled the tractor to dry ground.

This is the picture I have of God helping me when I got stuck in food addiction and emotional strongholds. It was a slow, steady process. I came out only because I was harnessed to the One who has the power, the One who knew the best path to take me to freedom.

## I WAS STUCK

I was stuck for years. In my mind, I was so buried in fat I could never be anything near normal. I could never have energy, clarity, stamina or focus. I could never achieve my dreams. I could never participate in normal, every day events. I was stuck in a prison of my own making and yet, I was in so deep, even God couldn't pull me out, or so I thought.

God had a plan, though, a simple plan to set me free. It started with me surrendering the things which had me bound. The plan He revealed to me back in 1977 is one I follow today.

I lost the weight, but there was still more God wanted to do for me. What could I do with all the emotional turmoil, anger and frustration still rolling around in my heart and mind?

It's like a giant puzzle with missing pieces in key places. I knew forgiveness was one of those pieces, but what was the source? That piece was necessary to complete the picture.

I needed to work on finishing the puzzle.

## ENDNOTES

1. Roberts, Richard, Patti Thompson, and Ralph Carmichael. Something Good Is Going to Happen to You. Light., n.d. CD. Psalm 34:4 NKJV
2. Psalm 34:4 NKJV
3. Psalm 37:4 NKJV
4. John 8:32 NIV
5. John 14:6 NIV
6. 2 Corinthians 5:17 NLT

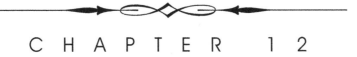

CHAPTER 12

# ANGER

*"God will break the chains that bind His people."*

Isaiah 9:4 TLB

I sat in the counselor's office not really understanding why I was there. After all, I was a rational adult. I wasn't crazy. However, anyone who looked at me could tell I had a really big problem. The nutritionist, one of those thin women who had never been overweight a day in her life, suggested I see the counselor.

I think maybe she saw me throw the food pyramid flier in the trash on my way out of her office. I'd tried those count-the-calories diets. They never worked for me. The counselor, though, didn't ask me about food. She asked me about my mother. Really, you want to know about my mother?

This was when Mom was battling colon cancer, and her prognosis was not good. I hadn't been able to cry or express any emotion regarding my mother's illness, so maybe that's what I needed to work on.

Her first statement was open-ended. "Tell me about your mother." It's probably a place she begins with all of her clients, but I didn't know it at the time. It just seemed she was reading my mind. In some way, feelings about my mother seemed to govern everything in my life.

I told her about my mother's cancer and also about her past emotional illness. I talked about how I stepped up to be the stand-in mother from an early age. I also told her about Mom not being able to come to my school events.

> Sure I had feelings, but I hadn't told anyone about them and I wasn't about to start now.

"How do you feel about that?" she asked.

"She couldn't help it. She was sick," I answered.

"As a child you must have had some feelings about that."

Sure, I had feelings, but I hadn't told anyone about them and I wasn't about to start now. Who knows what hidden doors those feelings might open up? No, best they stay closed. I shook my head and said, "Not really."

"Here's what I heard you say. She wasn't there for you. You did a lot of the work. She never supported you. She spanked you for things you didn't do. How did all of that make you feel?"

I dodged the question. I was supposed to honor my parents,[1] not be upset with them. My programmed response came out, "When someone is sick what they do or don't do is not their fault."

"Did you still want your mother to be there for you?"

"Yes, but I understood she was sick."

"How did her being sick make you feel?"

I sighed. Of course it did make me both mad and sad, but saying the words might make them real. I had been stuffing this anger all my life. I didn't want to "officially" acknowledge it and yet, I did care about my mother. The feelings were all tangled up together.

"OK, so here's the deal. I have so many different feelings it's hard to sort them out. I know how I'm supposed to feel now since Mom has stage four cancer. I just can't feel anything."

"Feeling nothing is a good place for us to start."

By the end of the hour, I had come to the place where I admitted I was angry with my mother for many things. I had always told myself I wasn't really mad at her. However, the more I thought about everything, the angrier I got.

## ANGER

Growing up, anger was not something I wanted to entertain. As a child, I experienced my mother being very upset and irrational. I didn't want to be the same. I began to see how I had been suppressing my anger. It wasn't a pretty picture.

What I really wanted to do was keep the anger and confusion about my mother from overwhelming my life. The counselor was helping unravel the protective shell I'd kept firmly in place so I could cope with and love my mother.

The lie I told myself was I wasn't mad at my mother for my childhood. I kept my negative feelings at arm's length. Constantly holding them off was exhausting work, however. It was kind of like trying to hold a freight train back. It was an impossible task. I needed lots of food for the required stamina.

At the end of the session, the counselor gave me an assignment. Before our next appointment, I was to write a letter to my mother using my dominant right hand. This letter was to be from the adult me, the person I was that day. Then, using my left hand, write a letter to my mother from the eight-year-old me.

"I don't think I can. I'm right-handed. I won't be able to read it."

"Just try it and see."

## THE LETTER

I went home that night and did my homework. What I wrote with my right hand was me telling my mother I was sorry she had suffered. I really loved her in spite of everything. I recounted some of the more important things, like how she loved and took care of my children and her other grandchildren.

I read the letter and instantly knew it was a real cop-out. It wasn't what I really thought deep down inside. It was what I wanted to feel. It was what my rational, adult mind knew was the correct thing to say, but it was not what I really felt somewhere deep inside.

I summoned up courage and began writing with my left hand. Here's what I wrote.

# DEAR MOMMY

I'm angry because you are treating me like a child when I've had to be the adult all this time.

I'm angry because you leave us sometimes to go to the hospital to get better, but you don't get better.

I'm angry because you never come to any of my assemblies, plays or other school events.

I'm angry because you never come to my mother-daughter teas or banquets.

I'm angry because you never come to my parent-teacher conferences.

I'm angry because you never compliment me on my grades.

I'm angry because I can't bring any of my friends home because I never know what kind of mood you'll be in.

I'm angry because you scream at me for ridiculous things which make no sense.

I'm angry because you beat me in anger.

I'm angry because I feel like I don't love you and yet, I love you so much it hurts my tummy.

I'm angry because you are not the kind of mother I want you to be.

I'm angry because I have to do stuff I don't know how to do.

I'm angry because you're supposed to be my mom, but I feel like I'm raising you!

As I reread what I'd written I was shocked. I didn't know I had all those feelings. I didn't like the feeling of anger rising in my gut. On the other hand, it was intensely freeing. I no longer had to keep these emotions hidden in the back closet of my life. I could own my anger. It could become part of who I was.

Facing my own anger was an interesting challenge. I had been taught anger was bad. To be a good Christian, I needed to get rid of anger[2] because it gives the devil a foothold.[3] I needed to put it away[4] and not let it control me.

Jesus was angry, though, and didn't sin.[5] He drove out the money changers from the temple with a whip.[6] He did it out of a righteous anger. Scripture also tells me to not let the sun go down on my anger.[7]

The meaning was clear. Anger is going to happen. I need to face it, understand what it's there for and either give it to God to handle or let it fuel me to right a wrong.

## SETTING THE LITTLE GIRL FREE

The little girl in me had held on to this anger past the point of adulthood. Even though I had begun to admire my mother for the wonderful grandmother she was to my children, I still harbored intense feelings of anger because of my childhood.

In order to set the little girl me free, the adult me needed to acknowledge how the little girl felt and embrace those feelings. I needed to begin mothering myself.

Being able to embrace the part of me which was angry was powerful. I was now a mother of two children, and I realized the ways in which they were probably angry with me. Using the anger I felt as a child, I was able to begin to be a better parent to my own children.

The action of acknowledging the negativity I felt as a child, allowed me to begin to feel other emotions. I was able to cry for my mother for the first time in a long time. The tears were tears of sorrow for the years I held her at a distance.

**The tears were tears of sorrow for the years I held her at a distance.**

I also began to face the fact I was losing her. In her struggle for life, cancer was winning. I grabbed hold of the hope of a miracle even when my mother surrendered to the fact she would not be on this earth very long. It was a bittersweet time. I had just begun to really love my mother, to truly understand many things about her life and the difficulties she had overcome.

Several weeks later, God gave me a poem about my mother's life. As the words came, I once again cried. I knew by the words the Holy Spirit had given me, He was revealing my mother would be with Him soon. I had begun to see her in a new light, and now our time together was coming to a close.

Sing, Momma, sing with the angels tonight.
Sleep, Momma, sleep in perfect peace and light.
You showed us a life lived for Jesus is a life fulfilled,
A life lived for Jesus is a life that is sealed.
Sealed for eternity in His loving arms,
Where struggles all end as we bask in His charms.
Sing, Momma, sing with the angels tonight.
Sleep, Momma, sleep in perfect peace and light.

There was more to the poem which reminded me once again of the phenomenal shift my mother's life took in the last 21 years of her life. Her legacy to us was one of an overcomer. She overcame her emotional illness entirely with God's help and strength.

## WHO MOM REALLY WAS

She had this incredible love for those who hurt like she had. She was drawn to anyone who had seasons of depression. She understood they needed love and support more than anything.

She would sit with those who were going through a bad time so they didn't have to be alone. It didn't matter if they talked or not. She understood silence is a language, and so is sharing the silence with one who understands.

Her very presence with them spoke of the fact they, too, could come out of the roller coaster they found themselves in because she had as well.

She loved her six grandchildren profoundly. I'm sad my daughter and niece, the two youngest grandchildren, don't remember much of their Grammy. Still I know when they get to heaven, they will know her. Her love will pour in a flood all over them.

Today, she would be so proud to know she has great-grandchildren. Her tribe is growing. She sits from the grandstands of heaven urging them on to run this race.[8]

The counselor left out one important thing regarding understanding my relationship with Mom. She did not say anything about forgiveness. In reality, I left the loop open. I embraced my anger, and I began to understand it was a part of the little girl in me who didn't really understand things.

Later, when I went on a journey to identify emotional barriers I had erected in my life, I wanted everything which would stand in my way of fully accepting the truth of who God was in my life gone.

I was having a really difficult time trusting the Holy Spirit. A spiritual coach invited me to picture who the Holy Spirit was to me. My picture was a confusing whirl of lights and sounds, coming and going, loud, then nonexistent. I couldn't reach out and touch Him because as soon as I did, He changed. The presence was huge, all encompassing, one minute and a wisp of smoke the next. Then, He would reappear like a screaming, howling tornado. It was very disconcerting and made me feel afraid.

## I CHOOSE TO FORGIVE

After the picture, I wasn't sure who the Holy Spirit was. It troubled me. My coach didn't let me stay there long. She began asking me to choose to forgive my mother for being confusing, for me never knowing what mood she would be in, for acting crazy, for being withdrawn and not present with me, for being angry at times and loving at times. I forgave her for making me feel afraid.

I did this simply by stating, "I forgive" my mother for each thing. My mother was already in heaven. These words of forgiveness were to set me free from the barriers I had erected with my own perceptions of what was going on at the time. I had allowed the barriers to be built as a type of self-protection. Now I was tearing them down through purposeful forgiveness.

As a child I didn't know better. I was an adult now. I wanted the walls gone. They were about to tumble down with one simple tool—forgiveness.

## COMFORTER AND TEACHER

Because the Holy Spirit is my comforter and teacher, some of the same roles an earthly mother provides, I renounced the lie that the Holy Spirit would treat me the same way I perceived my mother did. I renounced the lie He would confuse me, act crazy or cause me to act crazy, cloak Himself as something or someone I couldn't understand, be angry at times and loving at other times with me never knowing what I did to cause this. I renounced the lie I was afraid of Him and He wasn't with me.

This was huge. The relationship between how I viewed the Holy Spirit and how I viewed my mother was clear to me. Even though I knew I was filled with the Holy Spirit, I still wasn't sure I fully trusted Him.

I'd heard of some crazy things people have done in the name of the Holy Spirit. I didn't want to be a part of any such displays. I certainly did not want to be afraid of Him.

Then, I asked, "Holy Spirit, what is Your truth?" He was clear with His answer. "I teach you truth.[9] I lead you in truth.[10] I will never leave you.[11] I am always with you. You never need to be afraid. I'm always looking after you."[12]

The fact He said He would lead me into all truth was comforting in the deepest sense. It relieved me. I didn't have to be afraid of missing the mark or doing something wrong. Afterall, it could never be wrong if He was with me. He said He was always with me, looking after me.

"I just want to check something out," the coach said. "Earlier you talked about your picture of Holy Spirit, and in some ways it frightened you. So, I want you to close your eyes and picture the door of fear in your life. Is that door open or closed?"

I was shocked when I pictured the door. It was open and there was something in the door holding it open. "It's open," I said.

"Do you know why it is open?"

"My mother's foot is in the door." It scared me to even say it. I felt myself shaking. It seemed so real, I was sure the coach could see it as well.

"OK, don't worry. We can take care of it. We just need to go back and forgive your mother again."

I couldn't take it. My voice went up a few decibels. "All I do is forgive Mom. I've done this all my life. She was sick. I had to deal with it. I had to overlook it. So I forgave her again. I mean when is it going to be done?"

> Forgiveness is a process. We do it until it is done.

"Forgiveness is a process," the coach said quietly. "We do it until it is done."

So, I followed her lead again. I forgave my mom for targeting me for spankings I felt I didn't deserve. Many times children think they are being wrongly punished. This, though, went deeper than that. I felt I got spanked because she didn't like me.

I was bright enough to know I hadn't done anything wrong. This seemed to happpen often.

Possibly my mother was jealous of me because I would do her job when she couldn't. It left me in a precarious position, like I was between a rock and a hard place. If I didn't do the job she would be angry and yet, if I did it she would be jealous. This push-pull situation happened many times.

As a senior in college, I was home working during the January semester. My mother's healing was in process, but she still had times of unreasonableness. She began shouting at me about how she never had any money because they had to pay my college tuition. I had a scholarship, but they also paid a portion. I worked to pay for room and board. Many months they would send money to help with that as well. She said they just couldn't pay for the last semester of college.

> I wanted to please her, but she gave me no options.

I said, "OK, I'll lay out this semester, work and then finish next year."

"No, you won't. Everyone will know we can't afford to pay for your school. They'll know it's our fault, and you will blame me for the rest of your life." She was angry.

"Mom, if you and Dad don't have the money, I'll work and get the money."

"No, you won't. You're going to school even if we have to sell something to do it."

"I don't want you to pay for my college if you don't have the money. This conversation doesn't make sense."

I felt stuck. I wanted to please her, but she gave me no options. I didn't want my mother to be upset, but it seemed even the positive things I did, such as getting my degree, made her angry.

I shared this insight with my coach, and we went through the process again. I forgave my mother for making me believe I could never please her, for feeling everything I did, even the good things, turned out bad, for being afraid of her wrath and for feeling worthless.

That word worthless struck a real chord with me. I felt it down to the tips of my toes. I renounced the lies I can never please the Holy Spirit, He is not happy with me, He is angry with me and He feels I'm a worthless piece of nothingness.

When I asked the Holy Spirit to share His truth, His response was immediate. "I see your heart. It is worth more than gold to me.[13] You were redeemed by the blood of the Anointed One Himself.[14] Never forget your value in the Kingdom."

Then I saw Him like a warm and loving grandmother. I crawled up in His lap, and He covered me with a soft blanket. It was a place of comfort.

## THE COMFORTER

The connection was immediate for me, though at that time I knew nothing about the process. This was my very first experience. My mother was not comfortable to me. She made me feel uncomfortable in her presence.

One of the roles of the Holy Spirit is Comforter.[15] How could I allow Him to comfort me when I felt very uncomfortable with my mother? Instead, I went to a false comfort. I went to food, especially foods made with sugar and flour, which gave me a momentary high. I hadn't understood this connection before.

I knew Holy Spirit as Comforter in name only because I always went to what I falsely believed was a "sure thing" to comfort me. Food, though, will only comfort for a moment. The Holy Spirit is always with me, and will always comfort me if I allow Him to do so.

What I'm really looking for when I want comfort is peace and absence of worry and confusion. The Holy Spirit is peace, and He brings peace[16] into my life, not confusion.

"Don't worry about anything. Pray about everything. Tell God your needs, and don't forget to thank Him for His answers. If you do this, you will experience God's peace, which is far more wonderful than the human mind can understand. His peace will keep your thoughts and your hearts quiet and at rest as you trust in Christ Jesus."[17]

## TEMPTATION

When the session was over, I felt clean in a way I hadn't ever felt. There were still some areas I wanted to work on, though. One was this sinking feeling I wasn't totally free of the dirty, unhealthy habits of my past.

I knew there was a barrier of some sort keeping me from totally surrendering everything to God. I had been eating healthy for the most part. Only a few months before, though, I had succumbed to a temptation. At a conference I had eaten some gluten-free cookies, which had tons of sugar in them to make up for the other missing ingredients everyone had come to know and love.

My friend was the chef. She knew I ate gluten-free. She had placed little cards on various dishes on the serving table—gluten-free, vegan, etc. When I came to the cookies, which said gluten-free, I felt obligated to get a couple. I mean, she made them for me, right?

I took the cookie, and it was so good. I hadn't had a cookie in two years. By the end of the evening I had eaten six cookies, and had a bag of oatmeal, non gluten-free cookies to take home to my husband. This was a façade because my husband seldom eats cookies. Driving home, I had eaten two of the oatmeal cookies and started on a third before I heard the still, small voice speaking in my mind. "What are you doing?"

> Holy Spirit, is there a wall between us? Will You show me the wall?

God talks to me like this, giving me an option to learn from my failure. It didn't take a second for me to say, "I'm throwing this out the window" and then, I did just that.

I wanted to be sure I wouldn't return to this habit again. I said, "Holy Spirit, is there a wall between us?" I sensed there was. "Will You show me the wall?"

I closed my eyes, and I expected to see a shape that resembled a wall, instead I clearly saw myself trapped inside a chocolate tomb. It reminded me of the hollow chocolate bunnies I'd get at Easter. Only this one was about two-feet thick and hard. I was trapped inside. The wall was part of me.

I could feel myself getting anxious about this barrier. It seemed there was no way it could be removed without damaging me. I was intricately connected to my tomb. It was shaped like me, exactly contoured to me. If someone used an implement to hack away at the wall, I would be killed. If they tried to blow it up, they'd kill me. If they tried to cut it away, they would cut into me.

I would die if anyone tried to remove the wall, but I would certainly die if the wall remained. Timidly I asked, "Holy Spirit, can You give me a tool to tear down this wall without damaging me?"

I looked down at my feet and there was a large bucket of water. I instinctively knew to pour it over me. When I did the thick, hard-as-concrete chocolate wall vanished. I remained whole and complete.

## HIS PRESENCE

Immediately, I felt the Holy Spirit surround me instead of the substance which had held me back for years. Instead of a tomb of sugary chocolate, I was surrounded by Comfort Himself.

It didn't take a second for me to realize, I had just experienced the truth found in scripture. "God will break the chains that bind His people."[18]

I had allowed myself to be chained by foods made with sugar. This was a giant leap forward in breaking those chains.

"For the Lord is the Spirit, and wherever the Spirit of the Lord is, there is freedom."[19] I had God's Spirit. The problem was I had relegated Him to a small portion of my life because, even though I loved Him, I had been afraid of Him. It was exactly how I felt about my mother.

I'm sorry it took me so many years to finally forgive my mother for the things I perceived she felt about me. However, I'm so glad I did. Finally I could fully embrace the Holy Spirit as the real source of comfort in my life.

This set me free in a profound way. Now, I was able to begin to embrace my identity in Christ, a somewhat scary, but real necessity.

ENDNOTES

1. Ephesians 6:1-2 NIV

2. Ephesians 4:26 NLT

3. Ephesians 4:27 NLT

4. Ephesians 4:31 NLT, Colossians 3:8 NLT

5. Ephesians 4:26 NKJV

6. John 2:13-17 NKJV

7. Ephesians 4:26 NKJV

8. Hebrews 12:1-2 NIV

9. John 14:26 KJV

10. John 16:13 AMP

11. Deuteronomy 31:8 NIV

12. Isaiah 41:10 NIV

13. 1 Peter 1:18 NLT

14. 1 Peter 1:19 NLT

15. John 14:26 KJV

16. John 14:27 NLT

17. Philippians 4:6-7 TLB

18. Isaiah 9:4 TLB

19. 2 Corinthians 3:17 NLT

SWEET FREEDOM

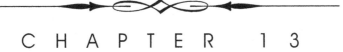

## C H A P T E R    1 3

# PRETTY

*"Behold, how beautiful you are, my darling.*
*Behold, how beautiful you are!"*

Song of Solomon 1:15 AMP

f I were to paint an abstract picture of Papaw, my mother's father, it would include denim blues for the overalls he wore every day except Sunday, the color of wheat for the fields he planted and the straw hat he wore, dark lush greens for the fields of clover, rich browns for the earth, bright spots of yellow for the twinkle in his eyes and the bright sun beaming down on his skin, weathering it and toning it bronze.

The picture would have a blurred, inexact look because of a specific thing he would say which always made me wonder what it really meant. Seeing him through adult eyes I think it may just have been a saying or an expression passed down through generations.

It was something he saw as humorous. It had always meant nothing of significance until I thought it might apply to me. For some reason, the comment unknowingly planted in my heart, seeds which damaged my already fragile sense of who I was.

I can see the picture clearly. I was about six years old. It was a late Saturday afternoon during the summer. Papaw was wearing his good overalls, the ones without patches because he had just come back from town.

He was hungry and was getting his special Saturday night supper of clabbered milk and cornbread. With all the great food Grandma cooked, I never could understand why he preferred to eat that.

> She may not be p-r-e-t-t-y, but she sure is s-m-a-r-t.

Grandma was standing at the sink washing dishes. Papaw was talking to her about a woman he saw in town. She was someone they knew. She had shown him where something was in the grocery store. He was laughing about it because he doesn't do much grocery shopping.

Referring the woman, he off-handedly said, "She may not be p-r-e-t-t-y, but she sure is s-m-a-r-t."

Grandma turned to look at him, diverting her eyes to me and back to him, as if to acknowledge the presence of little ears in the kitchen.

He got the hint, turned to me and said, "Did you understand what I just said?"

"Sure, Papaw. You said she may not be very pretty, but she sure is smart."

"That's right," he said to me smiling. I beamed at his compliment.

Then, he turned to Grandma and said, "See, this one's smart."

He didn't say it, but my childish mind filled in what he didn't say.

From that moment on, I knew I wasn't pretty. So, I sure better be smart or what else is there? I resigned myself to being unlovely, ugly and homely.

To me, pretty is something a person just naturally is. They are born with good looks. It wasn't something I thought I could work on, but I could work on becoming smarter.

Already school had become something I looked forward to. I loved to learn. I especially liked to read, write and draw. Tests came easy to me. I didn't have to study very hard. If I applied myself and studied hard, I could make A's. If not, B's came naturally.

I had adequate reasoning skills and could make good decisions. Being smarter became the thing I strived towards.

When I began to gain weight, it was just a symptom of what Papaw had said. I'm not pretty, but it doesn't matter because I sure am smart. He gave me something to focus. positive to focus on. I took it as being pretty just wasn't possible for me.

## SMARTER THAN SHE LOOKS

I hadn't thought of what Papaw had said for years. It really didn't color my memories of how awesome of a man he was. I knew he was just joking around and didn't mean it. Still, it was down below the surface of my conscious memory. I had no idea it was influencing me in any shape or form.

I had been married about a year when I went to work for a state denominational headquarters. I enjoyed my job there as a communications specialist working on brochures for various departments. Janice, one of my best friends, worked for a white-haired man with a dry sense of humor.

**I was trying harder to do everything I could to look smart, be intelligent and become successful.**

He was one of the department heads and one of the men I respected most. I worked with him to write and design brochures and posters to promote the annual meeting his department coordinated. Earlier that morning, I had dropped off the brochure for the two of them to approve. When I went in to pick it up, Janice said he wanted to talk to me.

He wanted to thank me for doing a good job on the brochure. He was genuinely appreciative. Janice overheard his words and called in from the other room, "He doesn't say that to just anybody, you know."

He answered, "Well, she's smarter than she looks."

On the way out I quietly asked Janice, "Is that a compliment or an insult?"

She whispered, "I guess it's your choice."

For some reason, I chose for it to be an insult. Immediately it triggered an association with Papaw's comment.

The adult me now believed the same thing the little girl me believed. I'm not pretty, but I'm smart. This reinforced my striving and trying harder to do everything I could to look smart, be intelligent and become successful. Of course, all the trying meant I had to eat more to try to stave off the pressure I felt I was under to perform.

Papaw, one of the most outstanding men in my life, condoned my weight gain. In some twisted sort of way, this became my reasoning as I put on the pounds. Now another godly man did as well.

I internalized their statements to mean I don't look very good at all. As a matter of fact, I'm pretty abysmal. Still, though, I've got the smart thing going, right? Let's go with that. I can do something about smart. I can read. I can take classes. I can become smarter.

It is difficult to ascertain how a person with any amount of brains could reason gaining weight to be a sign of intelligence. The pieces of the puzzle didn't fit together. Yet, there I sat, bachelor's and master's degrees in hand, weighing 430 pounds.

Why did it never occur to me if I was smart, I wouldn't be weighing almost a quarter of a ton? They'd be trying to do something about the issue.

## THE LIE I BELIEVED

It was clear, I had been believing a lie since I was six years old. Papaw's statement made to me in my childhood became something I perceived as truth even though it was a lie. I wasn't old enough to identify it as a lie and didn't know how to get rid of it. I took other similar statements and attitudes to mean the same thing. My emotional belief from childhood overrode my rational thoughts into adulthood. It was because unknowingly, I had continued to nurse and perpetuate the lie until it became my truth.

To deal with the lie, I had to forgive. However, forgiving Papaw was somewhat disconcerting to me because he had done nothing wrong. It wasn't what he said or meant, but what the little girl me wrongly perceived he meant and then developed into a full-blown life precept.

## WHO AM I?

Why did I take Papaw's comment to mean I wasn't pretty and could never become beautiful? Somewhere between ages three and six, I had begun to think of myself as not pretty.

When I was three, I knew I was beautiful. Everyone said so. Grandma had a studio portrait made of me which the photographer enlarged and set in his window. Every time we'd pass by it, Grandma would say, "Look at that beautiful child," and smile at me.

Then, I went to school and, all of sudden, I was larger than everyone in my class. When I look at school pictures I wasn't necessarily fat. However, I was always a size or two larger than most in my class.

I remember not being popular. I began the comparison game. I didn't have expensive clothes like the doctors' and lawyers' kids. I wore homemade dresses and things bought on sale. I outgrew my clothes fast. They never seemed to fit right.

I bought deeper and deeper into the lie I was not pretty and would never be.

My father and other father figures in my life set my identity by how they related to me and what they said. Dad emphasized education. He was the first in his family to earn a bachelor's degree from college. His degree was in Bible. To supplement the family income, he also worked as a steamfitter foreman, a job he got because he was the only one in that shop with experience and a college degree.

Dad reinforced being smart and getting good grades as more important than how a person looked. He was concerned with women who tried to "flaunt" their looks. He felt women should be extremely modest and not wear makeup or jewelry. When he gave compliments, they were always about intelligence or inner qualities.

I understand this. I understand he did not mean to make me feel I was ugly. He just wanted me to concentrate on what he knew would get me ahead in life and that was an education.

Given Papaw's comment, it is apparent where I got the idea it was better to focus on what I perceived I could change, rather than what I couldn't.

When I began gaining weight, I felt it was just part of who I am. I am a girl who gains weight easily. It doesn't matter, I'm not pretty anyway.

## RENOUNCING THE LIE

I forgave Papaw for the comment which made me feel I wasn't, nor ever could be pretty, and for making me feel I had to work extra hard at being smart. I also forgave my dad for never complimenting how I looked and playing down the idea I was beautiful in any shape or form for fear of setting me up to be promiscuous. I forgave both Dad and Papaw for never calling me beautiful.

I didn't need to forgive the older man who made the statement which triggered the memory. It was just an indicator I had a root issue which needed to be dealt with.

Because these were both my fathers, I renounced the lie Father God doesn't believe I'm pretty and doesn't want me to be. I renounced the lie He thinks being pretty is a sinful thing. I renounced the lie Father God wants me to work harder so I can be smarter. I renounced the lie He feels the only thing I have going for myself is my knowledge.

## GOD'S TRUTH

Then, I asked Father God, what is Your truth? He said, "You, Teresa, are beautiful[1] and intelligent.[2] You can be, and are, both. More than that you are My beloved.[3] You are Mine.[4] No one can pluck you out of My hand.[5] Anyone who says differently is a liar and the truth is not in them."[6]

Even with this one small act of releasing a misconception, forgiving, renouncing the subsequent lie this brought and hearing God's truth, I felt a sense of freedom in accepting myself just as I am.

In addition, I accepted it as more than all right if I looked pretty. I don't have to hide who I am under pounds of fat. I can lose weight and keep it off.

God revealed some even deeper truths in this area. In actuality I feared beauty. It took me years, but God set me free in this area as well.

## ENDNOTES

1.   Song of Solomon 1:15 AMP; Isaiah 52:7 KJV; Isaiah 62:3 KJV
2.   Proverbs 31:10 AMP
3.   Colossians 3:12 NKJV
4.   Isaiah 43:1 NKJV
5.   John 10:28-30 KJV
6.   1 John 2:4 KJV

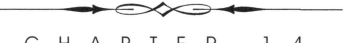

# PRIDE

*"The thief comes only in order to steal and kill and*
*destroy. I came that they may have and enjoy life, and*
*have it in abundance to the full, till it overflows."*

John 10:10 AMP

---

W hen I was five years old, I was convinced my mother was the most beautiful woman in the world. I remember sitting in the tiny bathroom in our house watching her put on her makeup complete with red lipstick.

Mom had acne scars so she wore foundation and powder. When she put on the makeup, it seemed she changed before my eyes. I loved watching the transformation.

She didn't wear eye makeup, but she loved bright red lipstick. With her dark hair and trim body to me she looked like a movie star.

"Mommy, can I wear some lipstick?" I asked.

She laughed. "You're too young for red, but maybe we'll get you some you can play with. Every little girl needs to feel beautiful." She ruffled my hair and then went back to finish her makeup.

She had just finished applying her lipstick when my dad came down the hall to hurry us along. He was preaching at a small Pentecostal church.

# FADING BEAUTY

He took one look at her and his face went white. "You need to take off the lipstick," he whispered urgently. "You can't wear red lipstick to church."

He left to start the car.

Her face fell as she began to wash off the lipstick. I was sad. Her beauty seemed to fade as the red found its way down the sink drain.

"Why does Dad not like lipstick? It makes you look so beautiful."

"He thinks being too beautiful is sinful."

"But why? God likes beautiful things."

"You go get your shoes on and find your Bible. We don't have time to talk about it now."

In the car, I tried to continue the conversation with Dad.

"When I get to be a big girl I'm going to wear makeup," I said.

"No."

"Why not."

"Because it's not what good Christian girls do."

For some reason that particular answer satisfied me at the time. After all, he was a preacher. He should know.

So, for the next 50 or so years, I didn't wear makeup. There were a few times as an adult I would go to makeup parties and buy makeup, but having not learned how to apply it correctly, I felt totally inept. I just used a little powder and lip gloss. After all, I was a good Christian girl.

## LOOSE WOMEN

As I got older, I understood my father's issue with makeup, shorts, sleeveless dresses, low-cut dresses, tight fitting clothes and even pants of any kind on women. He felt it indicated a woman of loose morals who wanted to attract men.

I had several close calls and run-ins with men and boys as a little girl and as a pre-teen. I determined I would follow all of my father's rules about what to wear and how to look so as not to attract any unwelcome advances. After all, I reasoned, any of the inappropriate ways males treated me must have been my fault. I followed all of Dad's rules except not wearing pants. In my way of thinking, pants protected me in a way a dress couldn't.

When I became a teenager, my mother began talking to me about boys. The feeling I got from those talks was if I became sexually active before marriage, it would be all my fault because I looked too attractive.

That's probably not what she said, but that's the way I interpreted it. With all the precautions and her feeling this would be something terrible to happen outside of marriage, I wanted nothing to do with being "sexy".

I did many things to make sure I didn't attract the wrong kind of man who might take advantage of me. There was a constant battle inside of me. Mentally, I knew I needed to eat healthy and lose weight. Emotionally, though, I found myself going back to the comfort of food any time I even approached a goal. I know part of this was the feeling of not wanting to attract the wrong kind of men even after I was married.

I've done a lot of work in this area especially in the last decade of my life. Even up until three years ago, though, I still wondered if after losing the weight there might be a situation where I'd start gaining again.

## FORGIVING MYSELF

So, I forgave everyone ever involved in making me feel like I might be leading a man astray if I looked like a halfway attractive woman. All of this was good to relieve a lot of emotional misconceptions. It wasn't until I forgave myself, though, that the big breakthrough really came.

What did I have to forgive myself for? Wasn't I the victim?

My own pride and desires were at the root of my issue. I didn't want to lose weight, wear makeup, style my hair, get my nails done or buy nice clothes because of my fear of becoming prideful. If I looked attractive, I might become filled with pride. Humility would go out the window. Of course, I knew the Scripture, "God opposes the proud, but favors the humble."[1]

I didn't trust myself to look too good. I might actually become what my father feared I'd become.

There was always this fine line I walked between looking presentable and yet, not looking too attractive. I could have just thrown a sack over my head and not worried about it.

Funny thing, that's pretty much how I looked in anything I wore when I weighed 430 pounds.

Forgiving myself for this hidden desire which seemed to loom so large I might have to "feed" it, set me free. I gave the Holy Spirit my fear of being prideful if I looked too good, and He gave me strength and peace.

## TIME FOR A CHANGE

Three years ago a mentor told me I'd be in front of people speaking and doing television interviews. I really didn't believe her, but I did have my first book launch party coming up. I knew I'd be on display there.

"Get your hair done," she said. "Learn to put on makeup. Get your nails done. Buy some new clothes. You need to feel beautiful so your inner beauty can shine."

I was 60 years old. It was about time I learned how to really look like a woman. My niece gave me makeup lessons, especially in foundation and eye makeup. I found an awesome hairdresser and a great nail salon technician. I bought some new clothes. I allowed myself to feel pretty for the first time in a long time.

I realized this is the real me. It's how God made me. I'm a strong, beautiful woman. I am not afraid. God's got my back.

Still I silently wondered how I would react if a man actually came on to me again? Would it scare me even if he was just joking? I was about to find out.

In April of 2015 my husband and I were on an extended trip for me to do several television interviews. We were eating lunch in North Carolina. I got up to go to the restroom and two men sitting with their wives or girlfriends at the table across from me gave me the up and down look. I could feel their eyes following me as I walked.

I noted to myself that they looked, but they did no harm and it didn't bother me. My husband was finishing his meal unaware of their stares. I was keenly aware my perspective had totally changed. I was not afraid.

## JUST JOKING AROUND

In Pigeon Forge, Tennessee, I found a gorgeous silver necklace I wanted to buy. The chain was 18 inches long. That day I was wearing a button front shirt. The first two buttons were open, but as I tried on the necklace, the chain was too long.

"Do you have any 16-inch chains?" I asked the lady. "I've been realizing my 18-inch chains are too long and the charms don't show with blouses like these."

A male customer at the opposite counter, turned around and said, grinning, "Just open a few more buttons. Problem solved."

Without missing a beat, I said, "Spoken like a man." He laughed, and I laughed. My husband had gone back to the car to get a bracelet of mine for the jeweler to fix so he wasn't even there to "protect" me.

In past years, if anything close to this would have happened, I would have panicked and fled thinking he was coming on to me. I would have ended up at the nearest ice cream shop with a triple dip ice cream sundae. My new perception said the man was just joking around and being friendly, not crude. I stayed, and bought two necklaces and a bracelet.

Somewhere in rural Illinois we stopped at a convenience store. I was buying a bottle of water. My husband was conversing with a biker outside the store.

I was paying my bill when all of sudden a man came up behind and hit me on the rear with a newspaper. Seriously, he did.

"Delores, aren't you even gonna' speak to me?" he said.

As I turned around he said, "Oh, I'm sorry. You sure look like Delores from behind."

I said, "I will take that as a compliment."

He said, "It was meant as one."

We both laughed. I walked out of the store smiling and liking the new lenses through which I was seeing the world.

## FEAR REPLACED

Somewhere in the last 30 or more years, both my perspective and my perception of men had undergone a radical change. It was a necessary change for me to be able to feel comfortable with my more normal body and not run in fear and hide behind layers of fat.

For years, I looked at many men through the lenses of fear. I was afraid of looking too nice and giving lecherous men the wrong idea. I know God allowed me to have these three experiences to show me most men are logical, kind and funny without any hidden agenda. I'm not sure why I thought otherwise. Growing up I had many male relatives, neighbors and church friends who were good men. However, the one or two I knew who weren't, tainted my view until I allowed God to show me I do not have to be afraid of men.

In the same light, I do not have to be afraid of being a woman. I am first a person and then, a woman. As a woman, it is more than all right if I am attractive. As a matter of fact, it is fine if I lose more weight. It is fine if I wear makeup, have my nails done and buy new clothes. Sorry, Mom and Dad, but it is also fine if I look as feminine and pretty as a woman my age can. I have nothing to hide, and nothing to flaunt. Pride and the fear of pride are no longer issues for me. I am free to be who God made me to be.

> I cannot be effective for the Kingdom if I am hiding, cowering in fear.

This is a 180-degree mindset shift for me. In 2013, I still wore fat-girl black-knit stretch pants and black tops because I still felt large even though I had lost 250 pounds. I still wanted to hide the woman I was.

When I began speaking in front of people and being interviewed on television shows with viewership potential of millions, I knew everything had to change. One day, I was still living as a super morbidly obese woman inside a normal body, and the next day I stepped into the life of a normal-sized woman who was on display for the world to see what it means to be set free.

This was God's desire all the time. I cannot be effective for the Kingdom if I am hiding, cowering in fear. He empowers me to be the best I can be. As a matter of fact, I don't think God minds at all if I put a little paint on this old barn. Yet, He still calls me beautiful whether there's paint there or not.

God helped me see that He replaced the fears I used to have with His peace. It's a peace which leaves me feeling normal. I no longer need to try to protect myself from being the woman I am.

Still, I am very much aware the fear I describe is the same fear thousands, maybe millions, of women feel. Many have more of a reason to have this fear than I do. It's a fear of what others might do to them, but it is also a fear of their own sexuality, a beauty so strong it naturally draws men to them.

Our society has made an idol of the female body. In some way, either overt or covert, sex is the selling point for every major advertiser. It's the tension between most men and women. Sex outside of marriage and the pull towards it is something godly men and women must guard against at every turn.

## ALLOWING THE HOLY SPIRIT TO LEAD

If I am sold out to God and allow the Holy Spirit to lead me each step of the way, I do not need to be afraid of my humanity. God made me as a sexual being. It is a gift He gave me. Used appropriately in marriage, sexuality, combined with an emotional and spiritual connection, becomes an intimate bond between husband and wife. So, why am I so afraid of this beautiful gift?

Of course I, like others, am afraid of the misuse of the gift, a burning desire we cannot quench. Temptation comes in all shapes and sizes. Jesus said, "Here on earth you will have many trials and sorrows. But take heart, because I have overcome the world."[2]

It is true, if Jesus could do it, so can I. He gave up His divinity for the time He lived on earth as a human with flesh, blood and desires. He was tempted in all ways like I am, but didn't sin.[3]

> The desires, temptations and cravings for anything which pulls me farther from God only control me if I give them control.

How did he do it? Many times Jesus pulled aside to commune with His heavenly Father. He had to go get instructions. He knew that as a human, His connection to the Father was what kept Him alive and gave Him power to overcome the pull of the world.

I have access to this same kind of connection to overcome temptations of all kinds. Jesus told His disciples that the Holy Spirit is the One who will lead, guide, teach and comfort them.[4]

The disciples were worried because Jesus was talking about leaving for good. They weren't sure they could carry on this Kingdom business without Him watching over them and keeping them accountable.

His reassurance was it would be better for them if He went away. As a man, He couldn't be everywhere at once. However, with the Holy Spirit it would be a different matter all together. The Spirit of Christ can be with all believers all the time.

The Holy Spirit is the same power which raised Christ from the dead.[5] Surely, He can take care of my simple desires if I will totally submit them to Him. The desires, temptations and cravings for anything which pulls me farther from God only control me if I give them control.

The Holy Spirit will lead me and be powerful within me, but only if I ask Him, only if I want Him to be. If I ask Him to He will begin to lead me, warn me and give me guidance.

Then, walking with Him becomes a marvelous adventure in abundance.[6] By His very nature, God's Spirit is a never-ending source of strength, power, love, peace and abundance. He is everything I need every day, every hour, every second to keep me from giving in to temptations of pride, lust, sexual sin, gluttony, envy or any other failure.

I was afraid of my pride, afraid of becoming too attractive. It's crazy for me to think one mindset sidetracked me in so many ways. Handing this fear to God, and hearing His truth that I am His, set me free in phenomenal ways.

I would need His firm truth, and much more, on the next step of my freedom journey, which took me into a deep area of fear.

ENDNOTES

1.  James 4:6 NLT
2.  John 16:33 NLT
3.  Hebrews 4:15 NIV
4.  John 14:16-17, 26 NIV; John 15:26 KJV; John 16:13-14 NKJV
5.  Romans 8:11 NIV
6.  John 10:10 AMP

SWEET FREEDOM

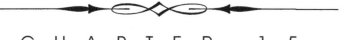

# C H A P T E R   1 5

# FEAR

*"You have a strong arm. Your hand is mighty. Your right hand is exalted."*

Psalm 89:12 NASB

I n 1994, I wrote in my journal: "I ran from intimacy with everyone except Roy and even then, I don't know if I can truly accept his love." It halted me when I saw it 20 years later because I didn't remember writing it. In thinking about it, though, I knew this was an honest statement stemming from being molested when I was 11 by a family friend, whom I'll call Fred.[1]

My thoughts and feelings have drastically changed since then. Now, I don't run from intimacy (both with my husband and my Jesus), I run towards it.

After discovering this journal entry, God dropped a statement into my heart. "Any disconnect with the one you are closest to here on earth will affect your intimacy with Jesus."

For many years, I still did not truly trust my husband though he had done nothing to merit me not trusting him. I had forgiven Fred, but I wondered if I was totally healed in the whole area of trusting Father God, Jesus and the Holy Spirit.

One day while I was running in the pool, I asked, "Jesus, do I trust You completely now?" I sensed I still had some hesitancy. So, I asked Him, "When is the first time this mistrust happened?"

There was a silence, a sense of nothingness, no response. I know when I ask any member of the Godhead a question and do not get an answer, it means I have a wall erected in that area.

So, I said, "Jesus, is there a wall?"

I sensed He said, "Yes."

"Will You show me?"

"Do you really want to see it now?" This time it was His voice speaking in my mind.

"Yes, of course. I don't want there to be a wall between You and me."

## THE WALL

In order to see the wall, I knew I had to close my eyes. So I went over by a tall concrete wall I could use to guide me as I walked with my eyes closed. They certainly weren't closed long. When I saw the wall, I realized why He asked if I really wanted to see it now.

The wall was an ugly, dark tangled mess of briars and vines. There were slimy snakes slithering around, poking their heads out at various times and locations. I so hate snakes.

My eyes popped open. I physically shuddered and began walking with long, deliberate strides. I asked, "How could this wall be removed?" It seemed impossible. It would take years to tunnel through. If He blew it up, snakes would explode everywhere, falling all over me. If He somehow buried the wall, the snakes would crawl out of the ground.

**Yes, My child, but it will take courage.**

I felt myself backing away from Jesus. Our conversation had been going so well, but now I just wanted to run far away. Trust, if it was ever there, had vanished. He would have to bring up snakes. I shuddered again and shook my head to try to get the image of the wall to disappear.

The inner healing coach in me knew I should ask Father God to help because He is the member of the Godhead I am most comfortable with. I asked Him, "Father God, is there a way to remove this wall without everything falling on me?"

He said, "Yes, My child, but it will take courage."

I smiled as I remembered my "I am courageous" socks I had put on that morning. I love how God orchestrates the details of my life.

I said, "Father, show me what to do."

I sensed He was telling me to reach out and grab the biggest snake, which was in the center of the briary wall, and pull it out of the thicket by its tail.

I hesitated and then said, "Father God, I will do this if You help me. Will You cover my hand with Yours? Will You protect me in this process?"

I pictured us joining together to pull the snake out by the tail. The minute the tail left the briars and vines, the snake and the entire wall vanished. On the other side was a beautiful, lush scene with mountains and bubbling brooks. Standing there was Jesus, my Jesus with His strong, muscular build offering His arm to me.[2]

I realized where we were walking was a place of trust. He and I had been here before, many times. I did not want the feeling to ever leave. I asked, "Jesus, why have I had a tendency to not trust You?"

## FORGIVING MY MOLESTER

I already knew it stemmed in some way from mistrust of men. Could there still be something left regarding the incident with Fred?

I did not tell anyone about that situation until I told Roy before we got married. He was supportive and understanding. Still, the fear of men who might take advantage of me was always there.

In the early 1990's I went with some friends to hear an up-and-coming Bible teacher, Joyce Meyer. This was before she was popular. There were only around 300 people gathered to hear her.

She spoke on forgiveness. She told her story of being sexually abused by her father for many years. Her story is 100 times worse than anything I ever experienced. She also told how she had forgiven her father and how that had set her free.

I had been internalizing fear of certain types of men, namely smooth-talking men whose words could not be trusted. I had been trying to protect myself. As Joyce talked, I saw Fred looming like a monster in my mind. I was a tiny speck and he was a huge hulk towering over me. It was the picture I saw anytime I thought of the incident.

> "Forgiveness sets you free. Unforgiveness keeps you in a prison of your own making."
>
> Joyce Meyer

It's why I tried not to think of it. I scooted it as far away as I could, but it stayed there as a controlling influence over my life. I could not get as close to people as I wanted. Something always held me back.

I mistrusted men. Any time a man would say something to me that even hinted of some sexual context, I would feel the fear begin to grip me again. I self-protected with food. It was a way to make myself bigger than the little speck I saw in my mind. Joyce's words rang true to me. "Forgiveness sets you free. Unforgiveness keeps you in a prison of your own making."

She explained forgiveness is a process. Simply say something like, "I choose to forgive this person for what he or she has done to me. I hand them over to You, God. Then leave them there.

"If they come back into your mind forgive them and hand them over to God again. If you are diligent and do this each time they come back into your thoughts, pretty soon you will think of them less and less. One day you'll realize you are no longer nursing the hurt. You are free."

She asked those who had someone they wished to forgive to stand and pray with her. As I stood, I saw Fred like a monster in my mind suddenly become a shriveled up little old man smaller and weaker than myself. Immediately I thought, "Why have I been scared of that all my life?"

Although Joyce said it might take many times to actually be free of the pain and hurt the person caused, it only took one time and I felt free from Fred.

## I realized the incident was not my fault.

A few years later, I attended a seminar where I learned adult men who sexually abuse girls or boys are called pedophiles. They don't just do it to one girl or boy, they do it to many. This helped me realize the incident was not my fault, although I had felt that way for years. The pedophile's issue, my age, my availability and my vulnerability all contributed, but none of it was my fault.

I didn't have to be concerned about hiding my identity as a female. The men who do these things to women or little girls have a warped outlook. I could not have managed Fred when I was a child. He was larger and stronger. My best recourse would have been to tell someone. So, I forgave myself for trying to protect myself when I was just a child. I also forgave other adults in my life who had no clue this happened to me because I was afraid to tell them.

The fear I was dealing with, though, was not the fear of Fred. It was something different. I had to go back further than when I was 11. That incident felt totally concluded, door shut tightly.

I had been off in my own world contemplating the past. When I came back to the present I realized Jesus was ready to answer my question of why I didn't trust Him. He spoke no words, but dropped a memory into my mind.

I was about six. Adam[3] was a year older than me. He and my younger brother played together. One day Adam said, "Come and play with us in our fort."

Excited to be allowed to play with the guys, I went to the fort which happened to be deep in some dense bushes. To get in we had to crawl on the dirt through a tunnel and then through a small opening. I already regretted agreeing to come.

Adam said we were going to play "doctor". I would be the patient and Randy would be the lookout. His job was to stay at the opening to the tunnel which led to the small clearing in the bushes, and alert the "doctor" if anyone was coming.

Adam had me lie on the ground while he used some make believe instruments to examine me. He lifted up my shirt to examine my heart. Then he said he had to examine all parts of me, so I had to pull down my pants.

Jesus was ready to answer my question of why I didn't trust Him. He spoke no words, but dropped a memory into my mind.

My mother hadn't really talked to me about boys except to say I was never to pull down my pants in front of anyone. Still, he was a "doctor" and we were just playing.

He began his examination which made me uncomfortable. I kept trying to get him to stop and telling him I wanted to play something else, but he just continued. About that time my little brother crawled through the opening saying, "Daddy is calling us for dinner." My brother saw what was happening, but said nothing other than, "Come on, Sissy."

## SUPPER TIME

I remember pulling up my pants and running home as fast as I could. At the supper table, Dad asked where we were and what took so long.

I said, "Oh we were just playing."

Mom asked, "Where? You took a long time to come."

Randy said, "In the fort."

"Where's the fort?" Momma asked.

"In the woods," I said.

"What were you playing?" In reality, I think she was just trying to make conversation, but suddenly it all turned bad.

"Adam was the doctor and Sissy was the patient. He pulled her pants down."

It felt like all the air was sucked out of our little house.

If looks could kill, I would have been shot dead by my mother's eyes right there.

"Teresa Kay, have I not told you to never let that happen? What were you thinking?"

I wanted to say that I was thinking of being a part of the group. I was thinking of having fun and playing. I was not thinking of doing anything wrong. I was only doing what Adam told me to do.

Instead I said, "We were just playing."

For several minutes, my parents just looked at each other. Then, my mother said, "We'll talk about this after supper."

After supper, she told me to wash the dishes and go to my room. Randy was allowed to go outside and play. She and Dad went to talk.

They both came back to my room. Dad said, "We do not want you playing in the woods with Adam any more. You can play ball or hide-and-go-seek around in the yard, but not in the woods."

"Does Randy get to play in the woods?" I asked.

"Yes, he didn't do anything wrong," Mom said.

Then, Dad left and Mom talked to me more sternly about how I shouldn't allow myself to be put in compromising situations. I really didn't know what she meant by that. She said more stuff which was over my head.

I was thinking of being a part of the group. I was thinking of having fun and playing. I was not thinking of doing anything wrong.

I pouted. It wasn't fair. I was the one who got punished when I felt it should have been Adam instead of me.

Several times Dad teased me by saying, "Hope you haven't been to the Pants Down Club today."

He was trying to make me understand he wasn't mad at me. Instead, I would cry and go to my room. He stopped teasing. I didn't want to think about what happened, so I buried this as deep as I could. All it did was bring up a lot guilt and bad memories.

Adam moved away a year or so later. I sensed my father must have had a talk with him because after the fort incident, he stayed pretty far away from me.

## THE DATE

Ten years later, when Adam was 17 and I was 16, he came back to visit our elderly next-door neighbors. I happened to be sitting in their backyard with them when he drove up. He smiled at me. He had grown up and was handsome. I noticed this because, well, let's face it, I was 16.

We talked for awhile, and I could tell he wanted to ask me something. I had to go fix supper so I excused myself. I had a Vacation Bible School program I was attending in a few hours. I was a teacher, and I had to be there for my class.

He stayed to talk with the neighbors. Before he left, he knocked on the front door and asked me to come outside for a minute.

"Would you like to go to a movie with me tonight?" he said. "We didn't get to talk much."

My mind hadn't thought of the Pants Down Club in years, but it immediately went there. I knew I should say, "No," but I found myself saying, "Yes."

Then the fear of what I had said hit me. "Wait, I don't know. I have to go to the VBS program at six and it won't be over until eight."

"Good. I'll pick you up at eight."

"You could come to program," I offered. Dad wasn't home to ask if I could go, but I knew if Adam came to church with me Dad wouldn't mind. I often went out with friends after church.

"Nah, I'll just pick you up at eight."

My mother didn't like the idea of me going on a date at eight at night. She hesitantly approved with two stipulations—get back by 11 and don't go to the drive-in theater.

Those days the only place teenagers could go to a movie after eight was the drive-in. I knew it, but I didn't say so. I was just too excited to have a date.

## THE DRIVE-IN

I was back to the house before Adam arrived. I was out the door without waiting for him to come in. I didn't want my mother or father asking where we were going. We left quickly, and sure enough, he drove to the drive-in.

"Mom said I shouldn't go to the drive-in with you," I said.

"And what do you say? I say I'd like to get to know you better." He put his arm across the back of the seat so it rested on my shoulder.

"I guess it will be OK if we're home by 11. What's playing?"

"Does it matter? I mean we have a lot of catching up to do. We haven't seen each other for 10 years."

"I don't like scary movies."

"I'll protect you."

He was right, it didn't matter to him what was playing. That was obviously not what he was there for. He was ready to begin where we had left off 10 years before only this time he was more adamant and more experienced.

## THE DAD CARD

At least four times I told him to stop. Each time he would say, "I know you don't mean it."

Desperate for a way to stop him, I blurted out, "I'm going to tell my dad exactly what you are doing if you don't stop right now, and take me home."

Although my father was not someone to be afraid of, he was respected by everyone who knew him. It worked. Adam stopped before he went as far as he wanted to go. Even with playing the Dad card, there were still some tense moments.

I was home before nine. He kept cussing all the way to my house. He was angry and kept saying he had paid for two tickets for nothing. I was just grateful for the nothing part.

The incidents with Adam were the root of the issue, but I was still unsure of how it connected to Jesus. It seemed more logical for it to connect to a protection issue, thus a Father God issue. I realized it was really Dad who protected me in both situations with Adam. Therefore, it could not be a Father God issue. That connection was solid. It was the Jesus issue—a trust issue—which was hindering me.

The beginning of healing the core of any issue is going through the process of forgiveness. In that process, the lies I believe begin to come to light.

Without total understanding, I began. "Jesus, I forgive Adam for misleading me, not once but twice, about his intentions. I forgive him for making me believe he liked me as a person and wanted my company, when what he really wanted was sex. I forgive him for making me feel guilty when he really was the guilty party. I forgive him for making me feel dirty and sinful. I forgive him for setting up fear in me which says I can't trust boys or men."

I continued. "I renounce the lie You, Jesus, will mislead me. You will take me places I don't want to go. You will place me in situations where I cannot make right choices. I renounce the lie You say You want to get to know me, but it's only to get me on Your side to use me for something to Your benefit. I renounce the lie You really don't want to be close to me, and You just want me to be Your slave. I renounce the lie in order to get Your attention, I have to do things I don't want to do. I renounce the lie I can never trust You."

That last lie was the main one. None of those lies had ever surfaced in my brain, but I saw how they were governing my actions of mistrust. The next question would unveil the answer I was looking for.

"Jesus, what is Your truth?"

As I listened to what He spoke to my heart, I began to feel emotions rise.

> The beginning of healing the core of any issue is going through the process of forgiveness.

He said, "You are My bride. I want nothing more than for you to sit at My feet, lay back against Me, and breathe and feel My heartbeat. My heart beats for you and for all of mankind, male and female, to be in close relationship with Me.

"You remember, I called John the beloved disciple because he understood what I was about. I entrusted My mother to him.[4] I only entrust My prized possessions to those I trust. I love you, Teresa, but more than that, I trust you because I know your heart.

"You remember My eyes search through the whole earth to strengthen those whose hearts are fully committed to Me.[5] Also remember that I see what you will be. Maybe you don't feel fully devoted right now, but I see your heart. I know when the rubble clears, your heart will beat fully with Mine.

> I see your heart and I know when the rubble clears, your heart will beat fully with Mine.

"Remember I have claimed you as My bride. You are My beloved.[6] I have called you to be by My side. One more thing, understand your husband is an earthly representative of what our relationship is and should be. Do not worship him, but thank Me for giving him to you. His strong right arm[7] should always remind you of Me."

I never realized before how much trust and intimacy are related. I thought again about the statement God had dropped in my spirit. "Any disconnect with the one we are closest to here on earth will affect our intimacy with Jesus." The opposite is also true, when we trust and connect with the one we are closest to here on earth that will affect our intimacy with Jesus in a positive way.

I know this to be true. I've experienced it first-hand both with my God and with my husband. It's almost too glorious to explain, but I would be remiss if I did not try.

## ENDNOTES

1. Not his real name
2. Psalm 89:13 NKJV
3. Not his real name
4. John 19:27 NLT
5. 2 Chronicles 16:9 NIV
6. Song of Songs 6:3 NIV
7. Psalm 89:13 NASB

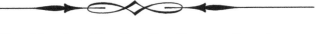

C H A P T E R     1 6

# INTIMACY

*"Step into life-union with Me for I have stepped into*
*life-union with you. For as a branch severed from*
*the vine will not bear fruit, so your life will be fruitless*
*unless you live your life intimately joined to Mine."*

John 15:4 TPT

---

Today, there is no greater joy for me than falling asleep in my husband's arms. I have been married since 1977, yet it feels like I just learned how to intimately love my husband.

I have always been in love with my husband, but I never really felt the level of intimacy with him I do now. Did losing 260 pounds make the difference?

Just physically losing weight is not the key to greater intimacy. The real key for me was losing the tons of emotional baggage I was carrying.

Whether that baggage came as a result of the weight issue or as the cause of the weight issue isn't really important. Discarding it was the thing which set me free to really bond with my husband.

As a former super morbidly obese woman, I saw myself as less than a woman, especially in the area of sexuality. I had reached a time when all of a sudden I was uncovered, exposed, open, transparent. There was nothing hidden.

For many women, especially those with any kind of weight issue, the message of skinny is better plays in our minds constantly. It's a message reinforced by any romantic novel, movie, television show and almost every form of commercial advertising.

> For many women, especially those with any kind of weight issue, the message of skinny is better plays in our minds constantly.

Many women have internalized this no matter their size. We just don't feel worthy of anyone's love. We can't believe someone would really love us if we don't look perfect. Of course, no one, not even the models, are perfect. Still, we are ashamed of our bodies and feel our husbands or any other man must be as well.

I was aware of the reality of how this played out in my own life during a television interview.

Arthelene Rippy, hostess of the Homekeepers show on CTN, asked me a question on a live taping of her show in July of 2014. The question caught me momentarily off guard. She asked if my weight gain affected my marriage.

Without skipping a beat, the answer flowed out of my heart. "I have the most wonderful husband in the world. He has loved me no matter what, and is very consistent no matter what weight I am. My weight gain did not affect my marriage to a great extent except that it affected me, how I related to myself, how much I gave to the marriage, and how I received love. Part of this [obesity] issue is being able to accept somebody else's consistent love in your life."

Once those words came out of my mouth I began to see how real they were. From day one of marriage, my husband has been the epitome of commitment, loyalty, hard work, peace, care and love.

For years, no matter how much he tried to show me he loved me by his consistency, care and attention I couldn't accept the fact that he really did love me. I would manufacture reasons to believe he didn't.

I'd take something he said wrong or out of context. It could be something simple that was meant as an observation. I would take it wrong and cry for hours over something I thought he meant which wasn't the case at all.

I put up emotional walls. I was afraid to trust. I was afraid he was just saying he loved me, but one day I'd find out he didn't.

> I put up emotional walls. I was afraid to trust. I was afraid he was just saying he loved me.

If I put up the walls then I could say the reason our relationship didn't work out was because I didn't want it to. It sounds ridiculous, but then my mind was so sugar-coated, any practical reasoning was non-existent.

The guilt about my weight always hung over me like a dark cloud. How could he stand to touch me when I didn't even want to look at me? I would avoid him, make excuses. I didn't want to be all in unless I trusted he was, too.

Years later, a doctor gave me valuable insight. "Your husband is like all men. We need to know we are making our wives happy. We need to know we are enough."

> We all need to know we are enough. We all need to know as a child of God we are loved, cherished and accepted just like we are.

The truth is, we all need to know we are enough. We all need to know as a child of God we are loved, cherished and accepted just like we are. Intimacy is as much about loving yourself as it is about loving another person.

Jesus gave us this truth in the Great Commandment. "And you must love the Lord your God with all your heart, all your soul, all your mind, and all your strength. The second is equally important: 'Love your neighbor as yourself.' No other commandment is greater than these."[1]

I cannot truly love another person until I love God and myself. How can I love God with everything which is in me if I don't love myself? How can I bond with my husband if I feel like I am not worth bonding to? This issue goes to our core. We stop at the outward appearance and don't look any further.

God does not look on the outward appearance, but on the heart.[2] If God's focus is on my heart, shouldn't mine be as well?

In essence, my outward appearance did reflect how I felt about myself. I wasn't sure I was worth the energy it was going to take to get healthy. When I changed my negative mindset to a positive one, things began to change on the inside and spread to the outside.

Having this kind of change helped me finally move towards true intimacy with my husband. This meant risking revealing my wants and needs. Interestingly, my emotional vulnerability laid the foundation for true intimacy to grow.

In the past, if my husband had a long day at work and was tired, went to bed, turned off the light, rolled over and began to snore, I took it as a rejection of me. It would set up the cycle of thinking I was inadequate because of my weight which would escalate into me taking inventory of all of my inadequacies.

Wait! Could it really be as simple as he was just tired?

We have come a long way since then to the point where we have learned to reveal our wants and needs to each other.

We share the simple acknowledgment it's been a long day, but tomorrow can start early. We know our love is a commitment we both embrace fully. We are even more bonded because of honest communication and total acceptance.

**Intimacy is not about an act. It is all about a relationship.**

Sex is an act any two adults can perform. Intimacy is in a totally different category. Intimacy combines the physical act of love with the emotional and spiritual connection which takes things to an entirely different level. Intimacy is not about an act. It is all about a relationship.

I have been happily married for 38 years, but I have been enormously satisfied for the last six years. Yes, part of it was because I finally surrendered my food addiction to God and began the healthy living journey. The other part, though, was because I allowed God to break down and remove the emotional walls I had placed around myself. This was another step on my journey to sweet freedom.

I stopped trying to be perfect and finally began to feel comfortable in my own skin. While it is true love is blind, at least to the physical aspects, love was not blind to emotional barriers I erected keeping me at arm's length from my mate. He knew it. He felt it, but couldn't really put his finger on the exact issue.

> I stopped trying to be perfect and finally began to feel comfortable in my own skin.

The problem was not within him, though I always focused there first. It was not about my exterior, though that was the next place I looked. It was inside me, and was buried so deep I was afraid to search for it. The barriers I erected for protection went up, in part, because of the negative experiences in my past with men and boys. Those walls kept both my husband and Jesus at arm's length.

Walls can't stand in the face of truth. It's just not possible. Truth hit me strongly.

My husband has always loved me. If some day we are parted, I know I will be the better for having loved full out, for having given him access to every hidden part of me, especially those difficult emotional parts.

It was this realization which became the basis for opening up, being real and connecting deeper.

I began with trepidation to reach out, heart in hand, feeling very fragile and way too exposed. I began by asking him questions and listening to his responses.

I apologized for my failures. I thanked him for the way he stood by me during my years of trying to eat myself into oblivion. He responded with care and love in a way which sent our relationship to new levels. Many times it was a hug, a shake of the head, or an emotional connection. True love needs no words.

Would it have happened if I hadn't lost weight? Probably not. The emotional barriers and weight gain were so intertwined it was hard to tell where one began and the other ended. The reality is, when I was willing to remove the covering of shame, guilt, anger and frustration and reject the lie which said I couldn't trust Jesus, truth stepped in.

**Walls can't stand in the face of truth. It's just not possible.**

I know I am loved, but more than that, I know I am worthy of being loved by both my husband and my Savior.

I asked my husband, "What has changed since I lost weight?"

He answered, "I can get closer to you—physically, emotionally and spiritually." I so love that answer.

While I lost more than 260 pounds of physical weight and tons of emotional baggage, I gained much more in true intimacy with the most important ones in the universe—my husband and my Jesus.

How much I am able to be vulnerable with my husband deeply affects our level of closeness and intimacy. The same principle applies to the level of closeness and intimacy I have with Jesus.

Jesus was trying to teach His disciples this in one of His last extended teaching sessions with them. He gives them, and consequently us, a word picture of what it means to be completely united with Him.

**Abundant fruit of the Holy Spirit is always available if I want it and act like I want it.**

"Step into life-union with Me for I have stepped into life-union with you. For as a branch severed from the vine will not bear fruit, so your life will be fruitless unless you live your life intimately joined to Mine. I am the sprouting vine and you are My branches. As you live in union with Me as your source, fruitfulness will stream from within you, but when you live separated from Me you are powerless."[3]

To be intimate with Jesus and to have access to His power, I must focus on Him. I cannot compartmentalize my life. All that I do must be done as unto Him.

Jesus said, "So here's what I want you to do, God helping you: Take your everyday, ordinary life—your sleeping, eating, going-to-work, and walking-around life—and place it before God as an offering."[4]

Jesus added, "But if you step into My life in union with Me and if My words live powerfully within you—then you can ask whatever you desire and it will be done. When your lives bear abundant fruit, you demonstrate you are My mature disciples who glorify My Father."[5]

Bearing fruit to me means to demonstrate the fruit of the Spirit: love, joy, peace, patience, goodness, kindness, faithfulness, gentleness and self-control or temperance.[6] Yes, I did have to bring up that pesky old word, temperance.

According to Jesus, when my life bears abundant fruit, all the fruit all the time, including temperance or self-control, I demonstrate I am a mature disciple.

The question is, "Why are mature disciples able to ask whatever they desire and He will do it?" The answer is because they know Him so well, they are asking with His heart in mind, not out of selfish desires.

When I do not want temperance, which means to be restrained in what I eat and drink, I am acting against the fruit of the Spirit. I have ruined my fruit crop at least for that moment. Abundant fruit of the Holy Spirit, though, is always available if I want it, and act like I want it.

## JESUS, MY INTIMATE FRIEND

Jesus wants me to be His intimate friend. It's really not that hard. Jesus told us how in simple terms.

"You show you are my intimate friends when you obey all that I command you ... I call you My intimate friends for I reveal to you everything I have heard from My Father."[7]

Obedience unlocks the door to intimacy with Christ. Modern culture says love and intimacy comes by going against the rules, running wild and free through the woods and hills.

My obedience to Christ simply means I love and adore Him. Because of that, I deeply desire to follow whatever He shows me. I do this because I trust Him. I cannot fully obey someone I do not trust.

It took me a while to understand when my husband asked me to do something, he was asking for a good reason, one which would benefit our relationship, not harm it.

God does the same thing for us. He gives us suggestions which are for our good, not our disaster, plans to give us a future and a hope.[8] Just because we can't see ahead to know how the suggestion He is giving us today will fit in with those plans, doesn't mean they won't.

> It's a life filled with humility. It's a life filled with grace. It's a life filled with complete surrender. It's the life I'm seeking.

We follow what He says, we obey His voice, because He is the Good Shepherd. We are His sheep. He knows us completely. We hear His voice and we follow Him.[9]

Why? Because we choose to trust Him, pure and simple. Lack of trust kills intimacy. Trust makes intimacy flourish. Jesus will not share everything He hears from the Father with those who do not trust Him. Jesus tells me intimacy propels me forward, not to self-acclaim, notoriety and fame in the world's standards, but to a life full of the Spirit.

It's a life filled with humility. It's a life filled with grace. It's a life filled with complete surrender. It's the life I'm seeking.

My life will demonstrate both peace and power when I draw on that intimate relationship with Jesus, the One who understands.

This is a truth I embrace in my life today. Each day I long to know Him more. So, each day I must trust Him more.

Here's what I have learned. At one time, I didn't trust Jesus. That lack of trust stemmed from a mistrust of how Adam, a neighbor boy, treated me as a child and teen. Not trusting Jesus led me to feel like I had to protect myself. I did this, in part, with consuming large quantities of food.

This lack of trust of Jesus spilled over to not trusting my husband. It hampered intimacy. Forgiving Adam, renouncing the lie that Jesus would treat me that same way and hearing His truth, set me free to trust Jesus again.

Trust became the foundation for intimacy with Jesus as well as for deep and true intimacy with my husband.

There are many benefits to losing weight and keeping it off. One of the deepest and most satisfying is not being afraid to trust both God and people.

It all goes together. Fixing the outside is not enough. Healing the inside is everything. Knowing God completely forgives all I've done is what seals the healing as done in Jesus' name.

## ENDNOTES

1. Mark 12:30-31 NLT
2. 1 Samuel 16:7 NIV
3. John 15:4-5 TPT
4. Romans 12:1 MSG
5. John 15:7-8 TPT
6. Galatians 5:22-23 NLT
7. John 15:14-15 TPT
8. Jeremiah 29:11 NLT
9. John 10:27 NLT

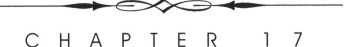

CHAPTER 17

# FORGIVENESS

*"But He gives us more grace."*

James 4:6 NIV

During a training exercise, I drew a circle, divided it in three pie sections and labeled them body, soul and spirit. I labeled from zero to 10 from the center point of the circle to the outside on each of the sections.

Then, I rated myself on how well I thought I was doing in the three areas. I gave myself a one on body. Hey, I was alive, right?

On soul, which I determined as my mind, will and emotions, I gave myself a four. I knew my will was sadly lacking. Emotionally I was being propped up with my comfort foods, and I knew it. My mind was what I always relied on to get me through. However, it wasn't doing a very good job of convincing the rest of me to get with any healthy living program.

Spiritually, now that was where I thought I was shining. I gave myself a nine. Me and God, we're BFFs. I teach Sunday School. I work in ministry. I attend church Wednesday and

Sunday nights and Sunday mornings. I was pretty good at this spiritual thing. However, how good could I be if I wasn't doing what God told me to do years ago in regard to eating healthy?

I colored in my pie sections based on where I ranked myself and answered the question. "If this circle represents how round the wheels are on your car, how far would you get?"

My wheel was sadly out of balance. If I had four wheels like this one, I would get no where. One side was almost completely flat and the other side was carrying the rest.

## WHAT'S WRONG?

Looking at the illustration of my life, I shook my head and said out loud, "This is not a true representation of where I am." I had felt my body was the main thing wrong. I was beginning to see my body was only the place where the difficulties were the most evident.

My soul and spirit weren't any better off. I thought my mind could carry my soul and my knowledge of spiritual things could carry my spirit. This just showed there was a lot more wrong than a few months of dieting could fix.

God designed me so all of my parts function together. All of me includes my body, soul and spirit. All of me has to be in line with what God wants. When one part is out of sync, my entire being is off kilter.

The Apostle Paul says, "May God Himself, the God of peace, sanctify you through and through. May your whole spirit, soul and body be kept blameless at the coming of our Lord Jesus Christ. The One who calls you is faithful, and He will do it."[1]

Every aspect of who I am is important to God, so important it should be sanctified as unto Him. He cannot sanctify or present me holy if I am still controlling parts of me. I must surrender every part of myself to Him.

Like all humans, I am flawed. I have sinned,[2] missed the mark and failed to reach God's standards. It's only when I give myself completely to my almighty God, I relinquish the title of sinner and take on the title of saint.[3] As a saint, I have hope of His calling and an inheritance of the riches of glory.[4] What more could I want?

I sat on the back deck of the lodge at the north rim of the Grand Canyon while my family was hiking. I just wanted to sit there forever and take in the glory and the splendor of God's majestic, vast creation.

**Many things look impossible, but with God everything He asks me to do is possible.**

The canyon is miles across. It looked huge. I thought of the song, "There is a cross to bridge the great divide."[5] The width of the chasm visibly reinforced the fact there is a wide gulf between me and God. There is no earthly way I can jump to the other side of the Grand Canyon.

Many things look impossible, but with God everything He asks me to do is possible.[6] He wants me to know I need Him. He wants me to know when I take a risky step of faith and jump there is no doubt His arms of grace will catch me. I am weak. I can't do anything on my own. I need Him. No matter how fantastic I feel, I need God more than anything else in my life.

God's commandments were not meant to condemn me, but for me to repent and receive this wonderful thing called grace. "Through the blood of his Son, we are set free from our sins. God forgives our failures because of His overflowing kindness. He poured out His kindness by giving us every kind of wisdom and insight."[7]

## Jesus understands the journey. He has the wisdom. All I have to do is tap into it.

Forgiveness washes my failures away and makes them as if they never existed. Grace gives me wisdom and understanding for my journey. Jesus understands the journey. He has the wisdom. All I have to do is tap into it.

I no longer have to keep a list of everything I've done wrong. I can repent, receive forgiveness and forget about it. He wants me to move on. I had such trouble forgiving myself it seemed better to stay stuck.

Throughout the Scripture, God says He forgives sins when acknowledgement and repentance is made. "Once again You have compassion on us. You will trample our sins under Your feet and throw them into the depths of the ocean."[8]

It doesn't matter what I have done. He forgives me when I ask. He throws my failures away as if they never existed. "The Lord is compassionate and merciful, slow to anger and filled with unfailing love. He will not constantly accuse us nor remain angry forever.

"He does not punish us for all of our sins. He does not deal harshly with us as we deserve. For His unfailing love towards those who fear Him is as great as the height of the heavens above the earth. He has removed our sins as far as from us as the east is from the west."[9]

This is really good news. For years, I knew what God wanted me to do in order to lose weight. It seemed impossible to me, and by myself, it was impossible. Yet, I continued to try to achieve this in my own strength with legalistic efforts at dieting.

I'm not saying specifics are bad. We need specifics, especially if we have overwhelming physical issues which require a specific dietary regimen. What I am saying is, God had the plan for me. It was an easy, understandable plan. He knew I wouldn't do a complicated system of points or calorie counting. It was a simple plan, but I made it hard.

I needed to understand He was not asking something impossible of me. It is impossible in my strength, but it is not impossible if He helps me. His grace-strength kicked in when I surrendered my self-effort. I cried out to Him, "I can't do this, God. I need Your strength."

> God's grace-strength kicked in when I surrendered my self-effort.

No matter where I am on my journey, I need God. I need His power. It seems He often reminds me of this by allowing me to come to the end of my resources. It is always His plan for me to ask for His help.

He knows I need His help, even if I don't remember I do. He allows circumstances in my life to remind me. To continue to receive the flow of His abundance in my life, I must continually tap into the power of God's grace through surrender. It is the only way.

"My grace is enough. It is all you need. My power comes into its own in your weakness."[10] God's power is always there in the forefront of my life. Grace brings power onto my life.

## GRACE IS POWER

For years, I didn't see grace as power. I saw it as a thing little kids get when they believe in Jesus. It's a children's song. It's not for adults. Ah, but grace is power.

It is the power to toss my sins and failures into the deepest abyss where they can never be recovered and are forgotten by God.[11] Sometimes I may remember them, but God says, "What sin?" He forgives me for everything I've ever done, even eating myself into oblivion. He does not heap the guilt upon me.

To find freedom all I have to do is hand Him my failures. I cannot go through life dragging tons of past failures, guilt, blame and shame. I just can't. I can't endure it. I have to stand in His grace-power.

"I know what it means to lack, and I know what it means to experience overwhelming abundance for I'm trained in the secret of overcoming all things, whether in fullness or hunger. I find that the strength of Christ's explosive power infuses me to conquer any difficulty."[12]

It's taken me a long time, but I have experienced the reality of this Scripture. I can attest to the truth that the strength of Christ's explosive power infuses me to conquer every difficulty. If I forget, I need only look in the mirror.

People ask me, how is it possible to lose so much weight and keep it off? I laid my weaknesses at His feet. In humility, I came to Him and said, "I can't do it, God, but I know You can and I will follow Your direction. You show me; give me the strength and I will go forward."

The fate of the rich, young ruler who went away sad[13] because he loved his money more than Jesus, reminds me even when God's directions are difficult, they are also right. When what He tells me to do is hard, I need Him all the more.

The clear choice for me became, do I want God or do I want a cookie? Do I want to live and serve Him or do I want to eat this cookie? That may sound like a drastic statement, but just suppose I am an alcoholic. Now, substitute "a drink of alcohol" for "a cookie".

It's really the same. Whatever I think I have to have, I am addicted to. Whatever I am addicted to, I worship. What I worship I put higher than God.

> Whatever I think I have to have I am addicted to. Whatever I am addicted to, I worship. What I worship I put higher than God.

When push comes to shove, my addiction will always win, unless I act against it. The only way I can do that is to submit to the power of God in my life. I simply made a decision to turn my will and life over to the care of God,[14] my God, the only One who has the power to deliver me from my weakness.

Looking at the lopsided wheel I drew, I began to realize a truth. If God is at the center of my life, He will radiate into all areas. I may never be well-balanced and free of my deficits, but

I can be complete in Him. He is the One who is all and fills all of me completely. I can never go wrong when He is truly at the center of who I am.

I handed my lopsided life to Him, and He began putting the pieces back together to make me whole, healthy and happy.

"So humble yourselves before God. Resist the devil, and he will flee from you. Come close to God, and God will come close to you. Wash your hands, you sinners; purify your hearts, for your loyalty is divided between God and the world.

"Let there be tears for what you have done. Let there be sorrow and deep grief. Let there be sadness instead of laughter, and gloom instead of joy. Humble yourselves before the Lord, and He will lift you up in honor."[15]

## BEFORE PICTURE

Several years ago, I was going through some old pictures. I found a picture taken of me at 430 pounds. I remembered feeling as miserable as I look in the photo. A friend suggested I take an after picture. I didn't really think it would show any huge difference, even though I knew I had lost 250 pounds and dropped 20 sizes. It was when I put the two pictures side-by-side the real remorse hit me.

I could visibly see what I had done to myself. I saw what God had been trying to save me from doing to myself. Yet, in my own willful attitude, I nearly ate myself to death. I did this to the physical body God gave me.

The words of Scripture ran over and over in my mind. "Don't you realize that your body is the temple of the Holy Spirit, who lives in you and was given to you by God? You do not belong to yourself, for God bought you with a high price. So you must honor God with your body."[16]

The guilt of what I had done fell on me like a 10-ton weight. It was only there a second before I did the one thing I knew it would take to remove it. I asked for forgiveness. God's forgiveness lifts every burden.

"Father forgive me for not listening to You. Forgive me for thinking I could have my cake and eat it, too. Forgive me for my stubbornness, for my pride, for the embarrassment I must have caused my husband and children.

> The guilt of what I had done fell on me like a 10-ton weight. I asked for forgiveness. God's forgiveness lifts every burden.

"Forgive me for causing them sadness when they thought I would surely die. Forgive me for trying to thwart the destiny You have for me. I surrender everything to You. I lay my weakness for sugar, flour and comfort foods at Your feet. I hand You my weakness. What do You give me in exchange?"

Not everyone has such a visible picture of the depths to which they have fallen, and not everyone has a visible picture of the victory God has won in their lives. I do, and I am so grateful for what He has done. So very grateful.

David said, "He also brought me up out of a horrible pit, out of the miry clay, and set my feet upon a rock, and established my steps."[17]

I love the old song, which is based on David's Psalm. It really expresses what God has done in my life and how I feel.

"He brought me out of the miry clay. He set my feet on the Rock to stay. He puts a song in my heart today, a song of praise, Hallelujah!"[18]

Oh, and what did God give me in exchange?

He gave me more grace.[19] He gave me sweet freedom.[20]

## ENDNOTES

1.  1 Thessalonians 5:23-24 NIV

2.  Romans 3:23 NLT

3.  Ephesians 2:19 AMP

4.  Ephesians 1:15-20 NKJV

5.  Point of Grace. The Great Divide. Robert Sterling, 1995. CD.

6.  Matthew 19:26 NLT

7.  Ephesians 1:7-8 GW

8.  Micah 7:19 NLT

9.  Psalm 103:10-12 NLT

10. 2 Corinthians 12:9 MSG

11. Micah 7:19 NLT

12. Philippians 4:12-13 TPT

13. Mark 10:22 NIV

14. "About the Alcoholics Anonymous (AA) 12-Step Recovery Program."Recovery.org. N.p., 29 Apr. 2013. Web. 01 Jan. 2016.

15. James 4:7-10 NLT

16. 1 Corinthians 6:19-20 NLT

17. Psalm 40:2 NKJV

18. Swaggart, Jimmy. "He Brought Me Out." Live From Nashville. JIM Records, n.d. Vinyl recording. Web. 01 Jan. 2016.

19. James 4:6 NIV

20. John 8:36 NLT

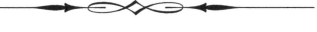

CHAPTER 18

# THE PLACE THAT GRACE BUILT

*"The Anointed One has set us free—not partially,
but completely and wonderfully free! We must
always cherish this truth and stubbornly refuse
to go back to the bondage of our past."*

Galatians 5:1 TPT

A reader asked the question, "Do you feel any different spiritually now that you've lost weight?" The easy answer would have been, "Yes". I have learned, though, questions are there to teach me something. So, I wrote a poem to help me understand why and how I have changed. Any change, especially total transformation is not easy. It's difficult, harrowing and simple all at the same time.

Jesus gave me the key to my freedom when I accepted Him as Savior. Along the highway of life, I willingly placed myself in a familiar prison when my freedom had already been purchased. Jesus never forced my choice, but choosing His sweet freedom was as simple as turning the key in the door of my prison cell. Then, I walked into the life He destined for me. I walked into "The Place That Grace Built".

231

Shades of blacks and whites
Long black angry shadows
Hiding fears, mistrusts and shame
And white as far as the eye can see.
Nothingness.
I wear my despair in monotone.
No cure for my sickness.
No help to pull me out of lifelessness.
No desire to climb to freedom.
Prison stripes. Prison bars.
Prison chains.
I am captive to myself.
I want to be free.
I want Someone to rescue me.
Unlock this bitter agony.
Set me free.

Silence is deafening.
I want to hear.
I demand to hear.
I know Someone is listening.
But no one answers.
Anger builds. Rage swells.
A fist raised to the sky.
Guttural anguish.
I want You to fix this.
I want to be loosed.
I demand an answer.
Ripping the stripes.
Pounding the bars.
Tugging at the chains.
It has to be easier than this.
How do I fix this?

A faint jingling
Could it be keys?
Could it be Someone is coming?
Could it be I will be set free?
He stops. He looks.
He weeps.
He turns to walk away.
Wait, don't leave.
Wait, You have the keys.
Wait, let me out.
His eyes bore into my soul.
Water and Fire,
Earth and Sky,
Birth and Death.
"My child, these keys are not yours.
You already have your key."

As quickly as He came, He left.
Though the words seemed a riddle
I remembered.
I knew the time.
I fell to my face.
I sobbed tears of regret.
I have lived my life for my own pleasures
And they have bound me.
I dressed myself in prison attire
And turned the lock myself.
I turned my back on His answers
Though He told me time and time again,
Surrender.
Repent.
Turn around.
Walk toward freedom.

Long, dark hallway.
Filled with perils
Leering from every corner,
Descending from every high place,
Grabbing hold and hanging on.
No, go away!
I am a child of obedience!
I am a child of freedom!
You will not capture me again!
Inch by inch. Step by step.
Choice by choice.
I am aware of a Power
Urging me forward,
The Wind at my back
Moving me closer to release,
Closer to the light of day.

Suddenly, there are colors,
Reds and pinks, Purples and blues,
Yellows and oranges,
The deep lush greens,
The brilliant hues of sunrise,
The dark browns of trees,
The grey blue color of my lover's eyes,
The bright laughter of my daughter,
The slow smile of my son.
Feelings return and I embrace them.
I no longer push them away
For the drabness of my cell
Is something I will never forget.
I know what put me there.
I know what will keep me out.
I never want to go back.

What I thought I wanted
Only bound me tighter.
What I said I wanted
Seemed too hard
To fight for.
I tried, I tried to get free.
Beat my head against the wall.
Screamed at the top of my lungs.
Tried short-term fixes.
In the end,
He knew I had the key.
I knew I had the key.
I just didn't want to go through the pain
Of leaving the familiarity of my prison.
I had become comfortable there
In the place of death.

The light of day
Seemed so far out of reach.
I could never go there.
Only beautiful people live in color
And yet the Creator made me in color.
He created me for better things than prison,
But if I choose prison
He will allow me to stay there.
Choosing freedom
Is akin to choosing Him.
Though I did that long ago
I didn't know what it really meant
To deny myself
To take up the thing that is my biggest difficulty
And make it my greatest mission.
To follow and obey.

Now, I know.
Nothing tastes as good
As freedom feels.
Those sugary chains
Look delectable, taste like heaven,
But they hogtie like hell.
I've been to hell,
I never want to go back again.
I've tasted heaven.
I want to do whatever it takes
To stay close to the One who
Inhabits this glorious place.
This is the place that Grace built,
A place of safety, security,
Beauty, love, power.
I live here now.

*Nothing ever tastes as good*

*as Sweet Freedom feels.*

*–Teresa Shields Parker*

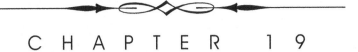

# C H A P T E R    1 9

# FINAL NOTE

*"The Lord says, 'Don't be afraid! Don't be paralyzed by this mighty army! For the battle is not yours, but God's!"*

2 Chronicles 20:15 TLB

I n the Final Note of my book *Sweet Grace*, my daughter said something I've been chewing on for awhile now. "I've watched you battle your demons for years."

It was in thinking through her statement and going on the next steps of my journey that I wrote this book. Still, I wondered, "What will she remember about my battles?"

She'll probably remember the times I gave in to foods, and the times I resisted. She'll remember the struggles I had with various diets. She'll remember it was difficult for me to trudge the short walk from the parking lot to her junior high school, and down the steps to the gymnasium to support her at her band concert.

She and my son will also remember I did finally learn to resist those foods with God's help. She will remember recently we went shopping at the mall, and had a great time buying clothes and walking though the halls. My joints gave out sooner than I'd like, but we did it and had a great time.

Through all of the battles I've faced, I've learned I do have an enemy. Except he's not the overriding power I saw him as for years. He only has power if I give him power. If I am unwilling to confront the issues which drag me down, I empower the evil one to continue to control me.

> I allowed the evil one to be the master puppeteer of my life for way too many years. He pulled the strings and I danced to his tune by picking up another candy bar.

I allowed him to be the master puppeteer of my life for way too many years. He pulled the strings and I danced to his tune by picking up another candy bar.

For others it might be a bottle of alcohol or some type of drug. On autopilot they hit computer keys which take them into pornographic displays infiltrating their minds and bodies. All the time, there is a kind,[1] gracious,[2] compassionate[3] omnipotent[4] God who loves them so much He lets them choose.[5]

I have never said to my children, "You have to love me because I am your mother." However, it has been my one overriding desire in life that they do so. I'm so thankful despite everything I've done and didn't do, they chose to love me.

The choice to love God is easier than to love an earthly parent. God is perfect.[6] He is a God we can trust.[7] He is a God who keeps His promises.[8] He is the God who sent His only Son that we might have life[9] and live in freedom.[10] But it is always our choice. He never legislates it. He says, "Choose Me and My ways. If you do, you will 'have and enjoy life, and have it in abundance to the full till it overflows.'"[11]

"Never doubt God's mighty power to work in you and accomplish all this. He will achieve infinitely more than your greatest request, your most unbelievable dream, and exceed your wildest imagination. He will outdo them all for His miraculous power constantly energizes you."[12]

I battled my demons for years. It was only when I stopped fighting the battle and allowed God to take over that real victory came.[13] It will not happen without His help and strength.[14]

My prayer is that my daughter, son and anyone else watching my life will remember my victory was only won when I surrendered everything to God whose power is made complete only in my weakness.[15]

That, my friend, is the sweetest of freedoms.

## ENDNOTES

1.  Psalm 36:7 NKJV, Isaiah 63:7 NKJV
2.  Psalm 86:15 NKJV, Psalm 103:8 NKJV
3.  Psalm 111:4 NKJV, Matthew 9:36 NKJV, James 5:11 NKJV
4.  Revelation 19:6 NKJV
5.  Joshua 24:15 NKJV, Deuteronomy 30:19-20 NLT
6.  Psalm 18:30 NIV, Isaiah 25:1 NIV
7.  Psalm 9:10 NIV
8.  Deuteronomy 7:9 GW, Psalm 12:6 AMP
9.  1 John 5:12 NLT
10. John 8:36 NKJV
11. John 10:10 AMP
12. Ephesians 3:20 TPT
13. 2 Chronicles 20:15 TLB
14. 2 Corinthians 12:9 MSG
15. ibid.

# SWEET FREEDOM
# STUDY GUIDE

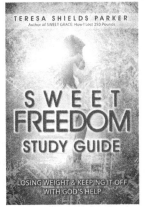

Now that you've read *Sweet Freedom: Losing Weight and Keeping it Off With God's Help*, I'd like to invite you to obtain a copy of *Sweet Freedom Study Guide*. The section on Inner Healing Principles is a practical guide to delving deeper into the emotional and spiritual portions of the weight loss journey, or overcoming any addiction. The *Study Guide* also includes Bible study, discussion questions and activities for personal or group studies to go with each chapter.

You can get a bound copy on Amazon or purchase a .pdf copy under the products tab at TeresaShieldsParker.com. The chapter she left out of *Sweet Freedom* is under the FREE tab. Check it out as well.

## WRITE A REVIEW

Please go to *Sweet Freedom* and *Sweet Freedom Study Guide* pages on Amazon and post reviews. With millions of books available any review long or short helps others discover *Sweet Freedom*. Teresa reads every review and says each one makes her heart sing!

# SWEET GRACE

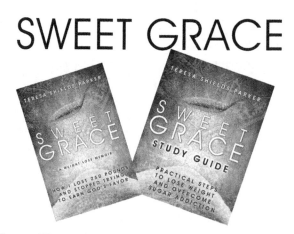

*Sweet Grace: How I Lost 250 Pounds and Stopped Trying To Earn God's Favor* is the #1 Christian weight loss memoir on Amazon. Teresa chronicles her journey of walking out of sugar addiction by the grace and power of God. She shares honestly and transparently about what it is like to be super morbidly obese, and what it takes to turn around and be free. Get your copy in print, kindle or audiobook on Amazon. Add *Sweet Grace Study Guide: Practical Steps To Lose Weight And Overcome Sugar Addiction* to use in conjunction with *Sweet Grace* for personal or group study.

*"Excellent, lovingly written. Brings hope, encouragement and insight. Highly recommend."* —Barb Thompson

*"Thank you for being vulnerable and allowing the light of God to shine into your darkest places that we might see into ours. Love, love, love the chapter on grace!"* —Luci Nicholson

*"This is the most inspiring weight loss story I've ever read! This compelling story of God's grace is a must read for anyone struggling with food addiction. I saw myself on every page and believe I have found both the physical and spiritual answer to my own struggle."* —Glenda Garcia

*"Life-changing inspiration for the person who has been unable to understand the life long battle with food. End the yo-yo dieting and grasp the truth of this book."* —Penney Anderson

# SWEET CHANGE

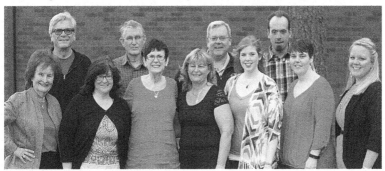

**Teresa, center, with some of those featured in Sweet Change book.**

*Sweet Change: True Stories of Transformation* is all about the power of change and how to tap into it. Teresa shares stories of individuals who've found their own personal ingredients work great with God's power in order to lose weight and step into transformation. Get your copy on Amazon today.

*"This book is amazing! On vacation in Mexico I couldn't put it down. Thank you Teresa for this wonderful and inspiring book of Sweet Change."* —Marjorie Eldredge

*"Teresa Parker has done it again. Her first book Sweet Grace opened my eyes to my own sugar addiction. Sweet Change is filled with real life stories of men and women who have come to that moment of realization in their own lives, and made those steps towards changing bad habits and ultimately improving their health."* —Anastacia Maness

*"True stories of true transformation. The kind that only God can bring through a willing vessel. Thank you Teresa for another inspirational book for those of us on a life-long journey of weight loss transformation."* —C. Turner

*"This book will inspire and motivate anyone to change their life for the better."* —Lindsey Summers

243

# FREE STUFF

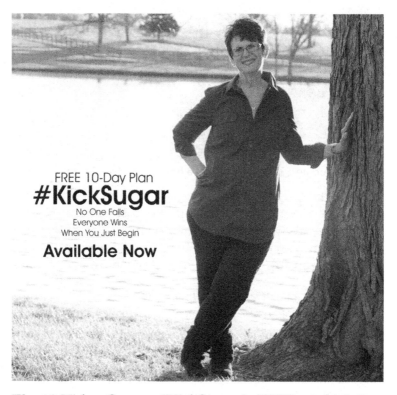

FREE 10-Day Plan
## #KickSugar
No One Fails
Everyone Wins
When You Just Begin
## Available Now

The 10-Video Course #KickSugar is FREE, and joining is simple and easy. Just go to TeresaShieldsParker.com. Click on the FREE tab and then on #KickSugar to begin your journey.

Check out the FREE *Sweet Freedom* chapter. It's the one Teresa left out of the book. She also has chapters of *Sweet Grace* and *Sweet Change* under the FREE tab.

There's much more on her site under the products tab. Don't miss the new low-cost coaching class #KickWeight: Essentials for God-centered weight loss.

## TeresaShieldsParker.com

# COACHING

Want Teresa's help on for your transformation? Sweet Change Christian Weight Loss Coaching Group is for you. You'll receive support, encouragement, weekly videos, action steps, accountability, monthly live call, interaction with Teresa, 24/7 group access — all from a God-centered approach to weight loss. It's time for you to become free and healthy — body, soul and spirit.

Go to TeresaShieldsParker.com/Sweet-Change/

*"Sweet Change group has given me a place to stop spinning in the midst of angst about needing to lose weight. I am gaining confidence I can change with God's help." —Carlene Coolley*

*"Sweet Change Group and the journey with Teresa Shields Parker is amazing and inspiring. Teresa's support, God's grace and the support of the group makes you stronger and reinforces your convictions." —Donna Barr*

*"I need a coach for direction and suggestions that work. I need the group to give and receive support. I need accountability and I love the spiritual support. I've lost 60 pounds and am nearly at my goal!" —Rhonda Burrows*

*"This has been exactly what I have needed to push through and continue on my journey."*
*—Heather Tucker*

*"Sweet Change awakened me to my special situation, and just kicking sugar for a few months resulted in a plateau-shattering 14-pound weight loss."*
*—Sharon Mello*

# IT'S HARD TO SAY GOOD-BYE!
## PLEASE STAY CONNECTED

**SUBSCRIBE** to Teresa's website at TeresaShieldsParker.com for ongoing blog posts and updates on new books, products and free stuff!

**FACEBOOK:** www.facebook.com/TeresaShieldsParker.

**TWITTER:** Twitter.com/TreeParker.

**PINTEREST:** Pinterest.com/TreeParker.

**INSTAGRAM:** Instagram.com/TreeParker.

**POST REVIEWS ON AMAZON REVIEWS** on any and all of her books.

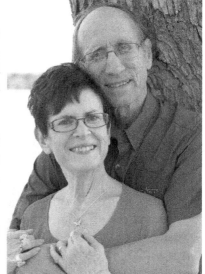

**INVITE TERESA TO SPEAK** at your group, church, Bible study, small group, Women's club, health fair or event.

**HOST** a *Sweet Grace* or *Sweet Freedom* study group in your community, church or club, and let us know about it.

**EMAIL** your questions to info@TeresaShieldsParker.com.

**Teresa and Roy Parker**

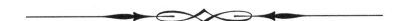

*"Never doubt God's mighty power to work in you and accomplish all this. He will achieve infinitely more than your greatest request, your most unbelievable dream, and exceed your wildest imagination. He will outdo them all for His miraculous power constantly energizes you."*

Ephesians 3:20 TPT

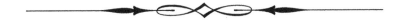